IMMUNE SYSTEM DIET AND RECOVERY PLAN

THE UPDATED AND PERSONALIZED PLAN TO BOOST YOUR IMMUNE DEFENSES, PREVENT DISEASES AND AUTO-IMMUNE DISEASES, HEAL YOUR BODY WITH ANTI-INFLAMMATORY DIET RESTORING OVERALL HEALTH AND GAIN ENERGY

ELIZABETH PATEL

within this book are for clarifying purposes only and are the owned by the owners themselves, not affiliated with this document

Page intentionally left blank

TABLE OF CONTENTS

INTRODUCTION
PREVENTION IS BETTER THAN CURE

Most Americans believe that health comes from the knowledge of doctors, not from our daily behavior. This strong belief is potentially disastrous. Every human being has its own goal: in life, in love, in friendships, in work, and so on, but let's remember that the most important is that of health. Every second of the day, our body fights to protect our life. A mechanism that defends us, a glass bell that repels all the enemies of our health; a mechanism that takes the name of the Immune System, and without him, we would not survive. Obviously, the functioning of the Immune System is closely linked to our behavior: the more we behave, the more he behaves well; the more we eat well, the more he defends us. Researchers from the National Institutes of Health and major universities around the world are discovering that a variety of foods, herbs, and lifestyle factors have a powerful effect on the immune system and, consequently, can improve your ability to fight illnesses. These nutrients and behaviors prevent disease and, in many cases, also help in disease recovery. Unlike the most prevalentdrugs, which exclusively treat the symptoms of the disease, the new immune system enhancers help prevent the onset of the disease. They also play key roles in helping the body stop cancer cells and cancers, even after developing. In addition to the most prevalentdrugs, there are also entirelynatural remedies that few know; moreover, scientists are discovering that many of these reinforcements have a substantial effect; for example, drastically reducing the chances of getting sick, some scientists confirm this - "... now we are discovering that in many cases there is a 50% reduction in disease and 50 % benefit from it".

For those who are already sick, some immune system enhancers can aid recovery and even prolong life. Among the most important are antioxidants, the nutrients that stop the degradation of cells and tissues that form the basis of many diseases and aging. "... .. If we could halve chronic diseases using nutritional therapy, we would make a big difference, especially if we consider the cost of treating these diseases": that is, almost zero, not considering the cost of the food you buy to feed yourself. Of fundamental importance, in addition to exercise and nutrition, there are meditation exercises and relaxation techniques that support the health of our body, also improving the ability to fight diseases. However, nutrition and exercise aren't the only powerful immune system stimulants available. Research shows that meditation, relaxation techniques, and other ways to use the power of the mind to support the body also improve the ability to fight disease.

Another fundamental aspect is to consider the health of our bodies today. We face new threats to our health daily, and we find HIV among the most dangerous. Other lesser-known diseases such as Ebola, to date, have not yet found treatments; for this reason, it is important to prevent these diseases with proper body care, and we will not be able to depend on drugs for life that will wear out our body in the long run. After analyzing old and new diseases, it turned out that the best defense is a strong immune system. Inside you, there is the most creative and formidable range of medical instruments ever conceived, at least when it is healthy. The health of that system is up to you. With this book, you will find out how to keep your immune system fit, healthy and strong, and improve health, and overcome diseases. You will understand the most mysterious mechanisms of your body. You will learn what foods you should regularly eat, how much physical and mental exercise you would need to strengthen your defenses. If you follow the advice you will find in this book step by step; you will simply live better. You will lead a healthier life; you will feed your immune system to defend yourself every day more against unpredictable attacks. This book will drastically change the quality of your life.

We cannot continue to base our approach to the defeat of diseases on external means, therefore through the use of drugs or surgery. Medicine has made great strides in scientific and technological understanding, but there are still limits and, therefore, diseases that are not yet curable, but in all probability preventable. Many diseases studied over the years, such as heart disease, cancer, or AIDS, have forced us to reconsider our approach and, therefore, today we are more focused on the need to prevent diseases before they occur. Hence, it is increasingly important to assist our immune system in carrying out its task of protecting our body. Over the years researchers have developed the ability to examine the system on a cellular and subcellular level, and there is now a deep understanding of the immune system and how it communicates with its trillion member cells, how its immune cells and proteins distinguish an external virus from its cells, and therefore manage to destroy these antagonists before they can cause more serious damage. And in a sense, our growing knowledge and growing technical skills have brought us into a complete circle with the first pioneers of medical science. As we delve deeper into the world of cells and chemical messengers, we face the body's healing powers, which we now call the human immune system. This book aims to illustrate the functioning of the immune system, to understand how to strengthen it by small actions of daily life and restore the health of your body.

CHAPTER ONE
HOW THE IMMUNE SYSTEM WORKS

The immune system is an arrangement of cells, tissues, and organs that participate in watching the body against assaults by "outside" intruders. These are generally microorganisms (germs) — little, sullying causing living things, for instance, microscopic organisms, contaminations, parasites, and growths. Since the human body gives an ideal circumstance to numerous microorganisms, they endeavor to break in. It is the resistant system's business to keep them out or, bombing that, to look out and obliterate them.

At the point when the immune system hits are injured or hit an inappropriate objective, in any case, it can discharge a downpour of ailments, including hypersensitivity, joint pain, or AIDS.

The safe system is inconceivably unpredictable. It can see and review a colossal number of different foes, and it can convey releases and cells to arrange with and get out each one of them.

The way into its thriving is definite and dynamic interchanges organize.

Countless cells sifted through into sets and subsets, amass like billows of bumblebees amassing around a hive and pass data forward and backward. When resistant cells get the caution, they experience key changes and begin to make amazing synthetic concoctions. These substances license the cells to deal with their turn of events and lead, enroll their colleagues, and direct enlists to burden places.

Self and Non-self

The way into a healthy immune system is its striking capacity to recognize the body's cells—self—and remote cells—non-self. The body's immune defenses ordinarily exist together calmly with cells that convey particular "self" marker molecules. In any case, when immune defenders experience cells or organisms conveying markers that state "foreign," they rapidly dispatch an attack.

Anything that can trigger this immune reaction is called an antigen. An antigen can be a microorganism, for example, an infection, or even a piece of an organism. Tissues or cells from someone else (aside from an indistinguishable twin) additionally conduct non-self markers and go about as antigens. This clarifies why tissue transplants might be dismissed.

In abnormal circumstances, the immune system can confuse self with non-self and dispatch an attack against the body's cells or tissues. The outcome is called an autoimmune disease. A few types of joint pain and diabetes are immune system illnesses. In different cases, the immune system reacts to an innocuous remote substance, such as ragweed dust. The outcome is sensitivity, and this sort of antigen is called an allergen.

THE STRUCTURE OF THE IMMUNE SYSTEM

The organs of the immune system are arranged all through the body. They are called lymphoid organs since they are home to lymphocytes, minimal white platelets that are the key players in the safe system.

Bone marrow, the sensitive tissue in the empty focus of bones, is an authoritative wellspring everything being equal, including white platelets bound to become resistant cells.

The thymus is an organ that lies behind the breastbone; lymphocytes known as T lymphocytes, or simply "Insusceptible system microorganisms," create the thymus.

Lymphocytes can go all through the body using the veins. The cells can experience a game plan of lymphatic vessels that eagerly coordinates the body's veins and corridors. Liquids and cells are exchanged among blood and lymphatic vessels, engaging the lymphatic system to screen the body for assaulting life forms.

The lymphatic vessels pass on lymph, a sensible fluid that washes the body's tissues.

Little, bean-framed lymph hubs are bound along the lymphatic vessels, with bunches in the neck, armpits, mid-area, and crotch.

Each lymph hub contains specific compartments where resistant cells collect, and where they can encounter antigens. Immune cells and outside molecules enter the lymph nodes through approaching lymphatic vessels or the lymph nodes' tiny veins. All lymphocytes leave lymph nodes through active lymphatic vessels. Once in the circulatory system, they are shipped to tissues all through the body. They patrol wherever for outside antigens, gradually floating once more into the lymphatic system, to start the cycle once more.

The spleen is a leveled organ at the upper left of the stomach region. Like the lymph hubs, the spleen contains explicit compartments where invulnerable cells amass and work, and fills in as a meeting ground where insusceptible securities confront antigens.

Clumps of lymphoid tissue are found in numerous pieces of the body, especially in the linings of the stomach related tract and the airways routes courses and lungs—territories that fill in as ways to the body. These tissues consolidate the tonsils, adenoids, and instructive supplement.

IMMUNE CELLS AND THEIR PRODUCTS

The immune system stockpiles an enormous arsenal of cells, lymphocytes as well as cell-eating up phagocytes and their family members. Some immune cells take on any individuals, while others are prepared on highly explicit targets. To work successfully, most immune cells need the participation of their confidants. In some cases, immune cells convey by direct physical contact, some of the time by discharging chemical messengers.

The immune system stores only a couple of every sort of the various cells expected to perceive a huge number of potential enemies. When an antigen shows up, those couple of coordinating cells duplicate into a full-scale armed force. After their activity is done, they blur away, abandoning sentries to look for future attacks.

Every immune cell start as immature stem microorganisms in the bone marrow. They react to various cytokines and different signs to develop into explicit immune cell types, for example, T cells, B cells, or phagocytes. Since undifferentiated cells have not yet dedicated to a specific future, they are intriguing opportunities for treating some immune system issues. Researchers, as of now, explore if an individual's undeveloped cells can be utilized to recover harmful immune reactions in immune system diseases and immune deficiency diseases.

B Lymphocytes

T cells and B cells are the principal kinds of lymphocytes.

B cells work essentially by emitting particles known as antibodies into the body's liquids. Antibodies ambush antigens circling the circulation system. They are frail, in any case, to enter cells. The activity of attacking objective cells—either cells that have been contaminated by infections or cells that have been destroyed by cancer—is left to other immune cells (depicted beneath).

Every B cell is customized to make one explicit antibody. For instance, one B cell will create an antibody that blocks an infection that causes the regular cold, while another enables an antibody that fights bacterium that causes pneumonia.

When a B cell experiences its activating antigen, it ascends to many enormous cells known as plasma cells. Each plasma cell is a production line for delivering an antibody. Every one of the plasma cells dropped from a given B cell manufactures a huge number of indistinguishable antibody molecules and pours into the bloodstream.

An antigen coordinates an antibody much as a key matches a lock. Some match precisely; others fit increasingly like a skeleton key. However, at whatever point antibody and antigen interlock, the antibody notes the antigen for destruction.

Antibodies belong to a group of large molecules known as immunoglobulin.

Various sorts assume different roles in the immune defense strategy.

- Immunoglobulin G, or IgG, works effectively to cover microorganisms, speeding their take-up by different immune system cells.
- IgM is effective at eliminating bacteria.
- IgA amasses in body fluids—tears, spit, the discharges of the respiratory Immunoglobulin tract and the digestive tract—guarding the passages to the body.
- IgE, whose regular occupation is most likely to secure against parasitic diseases, is the villain answerable for the symptoms of allergy.
- IgD stays connected to B cells and assumes a vital job in starting early B-cell reaction.

White blood cells

In contrast to B cells, T cells don't see free-drifting antigens. Or on the other hand, possibly, their surfaces contain specific immune responses like receptors that see bits of antigens on the surfaces of contaminated or cancer-causing cells.

Lymphocytes add to insusceptible protections in two critical habits: some quick and oversee safe responses; others direct assault tainted or risky cells.

Associate T cells, or Th cells, sort out invulnerable responses by talking with various cells. Some strengthen near to B cells to make neutralizer; others get microorganism eating cells called phagocytes; still, others establish other T cells.

Executioner T cells—in like manner called cytotoxic T lymphocytes or CTLs—play out a substitute limit. These cells honestly assault other.

Executioner cell arrives at the objective cell, readies its weapons on the goal, by then strikes —cells conveying certain remote or sporadic atoms on their surfaces. CTLs are especially significant for assaulting contaminations since diseases regularly get away from various bits of the resistant framework while they create inside tainted cells. CTLs see little segments of these contaminations watching out from the cell layer and dispatch an assault to slaughter the cell.

Generally speaking, T cells conceivably see an antigen if it is carried outwardly of a cell by one of the body's own MHC, or huge histocompatibility complex, atoms. MHC particles are proteins seen by T cells while perceiving self and non-self. A self MHC particle gives a prominent framework to acquaint a remote antigen with the T cell.

Even though MHC atoms are required for T-cell responses against outside interlopers, they, in like manner, speak to inconvenience during organ transplantations. Each telephone in the body is made sure about with MHC proteins, yet every individual has a substitute game plan of these proteins on their cells. If a T cell sees a non-self MHC particle on another cell; it will demolish the cell.

Like this, specialists must match organ beneficiaries with givers who have the nearest MHC beautifying agents. Regardless, the recipient's T cells will most likely assault the transplanted organ, provoking union excusal.

Typical executioner (NK) cells are another kind of dangerous white cell or lymphocyte. Like executioner T cells, NK cells are furnished with granules stacked up with incredible synthetic compounds. In any case, while executioner T cells scan for antigen pieces bound to self-MHC particles, NK cells see cells lacking self-MHC atoms. Like this, NK cells can assault numerous sorts of remote cells.

Phagocytes, granulocytes, and pole cells, all with different procedures for the assault, show the safe framework's adaptability.

The two sorts of killer cells kill on contact.

The fatal professional killers tie to their objectives, point their weapons, and afterward convey a deadly burst of chemicals.

Phagocytes and Their Relatives

Phagocytes are large white cells that can swallow and digest microorganisms and other remote molecules. Monocytes are phagocytes that course in the blood.

At the point when monocytes relocate into tissues, they form into macrophages.

Specific sorts of macrophages can be found in many organs, including lungs, kidneys, brain, and liver.

Macrophages play many roles. As scroungers, they free the body of destroyed cells and other debris. They show bits of foreign antigen such that it draws the consideration of coordinating lymphocytes. Furthermore, they produce an astonishing variety of incredible chemical signs, known as monokines, which are essential to the immune reactions.

Granulocytes are another sort of immune cell. They contain granules loaded up with potent chemical substances, which permit the granulocytes to demolish microorganisms.

A portion of these chemicals compounds, for example, histamine, likewise add to inflammation and allergy.

One kind of granulocyte, the neutrophil, is likewise a phagocyte; it utilizes its prepackaged chemicals to separate the microorganisms it ingests. Eosinophils and basophils are granulocytes that "degranulate," showering their synthetic concoctions onto hurtful cells or microorganisms close by.

The pole cell is a twin of the basophil; on the other hand, really, it's definitely not a platelet. Or on the other hand, perhaps, it is found in the lungs, skin, tongue, and linings of the nose and intestinal tract, where it is obligated for the manifestations of sensitivity.

A related structure, the blood platelet, is a cell part. Platelets, as well, contain granules. Notwithstanding advancing blood thickening and wound fix, platelets initiate a portion of the immune defenses.

Cytokines

Segments of the immune system speak with each other by trading chemical messengers called cytokines. These proteins are discharged by cells and follow up on different cells to facilitate a suitable immune reaction. Cytokines fuse different assortment of interleukins, interferons, and development factors.

A couple of cytokines are concoction switches that turn certain insusceptible cell types on and off.

One cytokine, interleukin 2 (IL-2), triggers the resistant framework to convey T cells. IL2's resistance boosting properties have generally made it a promising treatment for a couple of afflictions. Clinical specialists are advancing to test their preferences in various sicknesses, for instance, malignancy, hepatitis C, and HIV ailment and AIDS. Various cytokines in like manner are being read for their potential clinical preferred position. Different cytokines chemically draw in explicit cell types. These supposed chemokines are discharged by cells at a site of injury or disease and consider other immune cells to the region to help fix the harm or ward off the intruder. Chemokine regularly assumes a key job in inflammation and is a promising objective for new medications to help direct immune reactions.

Complement

The complement system is comprised of around 25 proteins that cooperate to "complement" the activity of antibodies in devastating microscopic organisms. Complement additionally assists with freeing the body of antibody-coated antigens (antigen-immune response edifices). Complement proteins, which cause veins to become expanded and afterward cracked, add to the redness, warmth, growing, pain, and loss of capacity that describe a provocative reaction.

Complement proteins flow in the blood in a latent structure. At the point when the primary protein in the complement series is actuated—regularly by an immune response that has bolted onto an antigen—it gets a domino impact underway. Every segment proceeds in an exact chain of steps known as the complement course. The finished result is a cylinder inserted into—and puncturing an opening in—the cell's divider. With liquids and molecules streaming in and out, the cell swells and blasts. Different parts of the complement system make microorganisms progressively defenseless to phagocytosis or entice different cells to the area.

Mounting an Immune Response

Infections are the most well-known reason for human illness. They run from the normal cold to incapacitating conditions like ceaseless hepatitis to dangerous diseases, for example, AIDS. Illness causing microorganisms (pathogens) endeavoring to get into the body should initially move past the body's outer covering, typically the skin or cells coating the body's inside ways.

The skin gives an overwhelming hindrance to attacking microorganisms. It is commonly vulnerable just through cuts or minor scraped places. The digestive and respiratory tracts—the two portals of passage for various microorganisms—additionally have their degrees of assurance. Organisms entering the nose regularly cause the nasal surfaces to emit increasingly defensive bodily fluid, and endeavors to enter the nose or lungs can trigger a sniffle or chop reflex to compel microbial trespassers out of the respiratory paths. The stomach contains a healthy corrosive that annihilates many pathogens that are swallowed with food.

If microorganisms endure the body's bleeding-edge immunity, they, despite everything, need to discover a way through the walls of the stomach related, respiratory, or urogenital paths to the hidden cells. These paths are fixed with firmly stuffed epithelial cells canvassed in a mucus layer, successfully hindering the vehicle of many organisms.

Mucosal surfaces likewise discharge an extraordinary class of antibodies called IgA, which, much of the time, is the primary kind of immunizer to experience an attacking microorganism.

Underneath the epithelial layer, various cells, including macrophages, B cells, and T cells, lie in sit tight for any germ that may bypass the boundaries at the surface.

Next, intruders must get away from a progression of general protections prepared to attack, without respect for explicit antigen markers: these incorporate watching phagocytes, NK cells, and complement.

Microbes that cross the general obstructions at that point go up against specific weapons custom fitted only for them. Explicit weapons, which incorporate the two antibodies and T cells, are outfitted with particular receptor structures that permit them to perceive and connect with their designated targets.

Bacteria, Viruses, and Parasites

The most widely recognized infection-causing microbes are bacteria and parasites. Every utilization of an alternate strategy to contaminate an individual, and, in this way, each is defeated by an alternate piece of the immune system.

Most bacteria live inside the spaces among cells and are promptly attacked by antibodies. At the point when antibodies connect to a bacterium, they impart signs to complement phagocytic cells and proteins to destroy the bound microorganisms. A few microscopic organisms are eaten straightforwardly by phagocytes, which signify certain T cells to join the attack.

All viruses, in addition to a couple of sorts of microscopic organisms and parasites, must enter cells to endure, requiring an alternate methodology. Tainted cells utilize their MHC molecules to put bits of the attacking organisms on the phone's surface, waving to cytotoxic T lymphocytes to demolish the contaminated cell Antibodies additionally can aid the immune reaction, connecting to and clearing infections before they get an opportunity to enter the cell.

Parasites live either inside or outside cells. Intracellular parasites, for example, the life form that causes malaria can trigger T-cell reactions. Extracellular parasites are frequently a lot bigger than bacteria organisms or infections and require a lot more extensive immune attack. Parasitic Infections regularly trigger an incendiary reaction when eosinophils, basophils, and other particular granular cells race to the scene and discharge their stores of poisonous chemicals substances trying to demolish the trespasser. Antibodies also assume a job in this attack, drawing the granular cells to the site of infection.

Invulnerability: Natural and Acquired

In the past, doctors understood that individuals who had recouped from the plague could never get it again—they had gained immunity. This is because a portion of the enacted T and B cells become memory cells.

Whenever an individual gets together with a similar antigen, the immune system is set to annihilate it.

Immunity can be healthy or powerless, short-lived or enduring, contingent upon the sort of antigen, the measure of antigen, and the course by which it enters the body.

Immunity can likewise be affected by acquired qualities. When confronted with a similar antigen, a few people will react compellingly, others weakly, and some are not under any condition.

An immune reaction can be started by disease as well as by vaccination with antibodies. Vaccines contain microorganisms— or parts of microorganisms—that have been dealt with so they can incite an immune reaction yet not all out disease.

Immunity can likewise be moved to start with one individual then onto the next by infusions of serum wealthy in antibodies against a specific organism (antiserum).

For instance, the immune serum is now and again given to protect travelers to nations where hepatitis A is boundless. Such aloof immunity regularly endures just half a month or months.

Newborn children are brought into the world with weak immune reactions; however, are secured for the initial hardly any long periods of life by antibodies got from their moms before birth. Infants who are breastfed can likewise get a few antibodies from bosom milk that helps to ensure their stomach related tracts.

Immune Tolerance

Immune tolerance is the propensity of T or B lymphocytes to overlook the body's tissues. Keeping up immunity is significant because it keeps the immune system from attacking its fellow cells. Researchers are working diligently attempting to see how the immune system realizes when to react and when to ignore it.

Tolerance occurs in at least two ways.

Central tolerance happens during lymphocyte advancement. Early in every immune cell's life, it is presented to a large number of the self-molecules in the body. If it experiences these molecules before it has completely developed, it actuates an inward fall to pieces pathway, and the immune cell dies. This procedure, called clonal erasure, guarantees that self-reactive T cells and B cells don't develop and attack healthy tissues.

Since developing lymphocytes don't experience each molecule in the body, they should likewise figure out how to disregard develop cells and tissues. Infringe tolerance, circling lymphocytes may perceive a self-molecule yet can't react because a portion of the chemical signs required to actuate the T or B cell is missing. Purported clonal energy, thusly, keeps conceivably harmful lymphocytes turned off. Fringe tolerance may likewise be forced by an uncommon class of administrative T cells that restrains assistant or cytotoxic T-cell activation by self-antigens.

Vaccines

Since a while ago, medical workers have helped the body's immune system get ready for future attacks through vaccination. Vaccines comprise of killed or adjusted microorganisms, segments of organisms, or microbial DNA that trick the body into intuition contamination has happened. A vaccinated individual's immune system attacks the innocuous immunization and gets ready for ensuing intrusions. Vaccines stay probably the ideal approaches to forestall irresistible diseases and have a magnificent health record. Already annihilating illnesses, such as smallpox, polio, and challenging chop, have been extraordinarily controlled or dispensed with through overall immunization programs.

Disorders of the Immune System

Allergic Diseases

The most widely recognized sorts of allergic diseases happen when the immune system reacts to a false alarm. In an allergic individual, a typically innocuous material, like grass dust or house dust, is confused with danger and attacked.

Allergies, for example, dust allergy, are identified with the antibody known as IgE. Like different antibodies, every IgE antibody is explicit; one acts against oak pollen, another against ragweed.

Immune system Diseases sometimes, the immune system's acknowledgment contraption separates, and the body starts to manufacture antibodies and T cells coordinated against its cells and organs. Confused autoantibodies and T cells, as they are known, add too many diseases. For example, Lymphocytes which assault pancreas cells add to diabetes, while an autoantibody known as a rheumatoid factor is ordinary in people with rheumatoid joint torment. Individuals with fundamental lupus erythematosus (SLE) have Antibodies to many sorts of their cells and cell parts.

Nobody knows precisely what causes an immune system sickness, yet different elements will probably be included. These remember components for the earth, for example, infections, certain medications, and daylight, all of which may harm or modify typical body cells. Hormones are associated with playing a role since most immune system infections are more typical in ladies than in men.

Heredity, too, is by all accounts in any way significant.

Many individuals with immune system illnesses have trademark sorts of self-marker molecules.

Immune Complex Diseases

Immune buildings are groups of interlocking antigens and antibodies.

Regularly, immune buildings are quickly expelled from the bloodstream. Here and there, in any case, they proceed to course, and in the long run, become trapped in the tissues of the kidneys, the lungs, skin, joints, or veins. There they set off responses with a complement that leads to inflammation and tissue harm.

Immune complexes work their mischief in many diseases. These incorporate intestinal sickness and viral hepatitis, just as many immune system diseases.

Immunodeficiency Disorders

When the immune system is missing at least one of its parts, the outcome is an immunodeficiency disorder.

Immunodeficiency disorders can be acquired, gained through disease, or created unexpectedly by medications, for example, those used to treat individuals with cancer or the individuals who have gotten transplants.

Temporary immune insufficiencies can create in the wake of regular virus Infections, including flu, irresistible mononucleosis, and measles. Likewise, immune reactions can be discouraged by blood transfusions, medical procedures, ailing health, smoking, and stress.

A few youngsters are brought into the world with ineffectively working immune systems. Some have defects in the B cell system and can't create antibodies. Others, whose thymus is either absent or small and unusual, need T cells. Rarely, babies are born lacking all of the entirety of the significant immune defenses.

This condition is known as extreme joined immunodeficiency disease or SCID.

AIDS is an immunodeficiency issue brought about by an infection (HIV) that contaminates immune cells. HIV can crush or handicap indispensable T cells, making ready for a variety of immunologic inadequacies. HIV likewise can hang out for significant stretches in immune cells. As the immune defenses vacillate, an individual with AIDS falls prey to abnormal, regularly dangerous Infections and uncommon diseases.

An infectious disease, AIDS is spread by close sexual contact, move of the infection from mother to newborn child during pregnancy, or direct blood tainting.

There is no remedy for AIDS, however recently created antiviral medications can slow the development of the disease, at any rate for a period.

Researchers likewise are trying HIV vaccines in clinical studies.

CANCERS OF THE IMMUNE SYSTEM

The cells of the immune system, as different cells, can develop wildly, bringing about cancer. Leukemia is brought about by the multiplication of white blood cells, or leukocytes. The uncontrolled development of antibody delivering plasma cells can prompt different myeloma. Cancers of the lymphoid organs, known as lymphomas, incorporate Hodgkin's illness.

Immunology and Transplants

Consistently an enormous number of American lives are drawn out by transplanted organs—kidney, heart, lung, liver, and pancreas. For a transplant to "take," regardless, the body's basic tendency to free itself of outside tissue must be repealed.

One way, tissue creating, guarantees markers of self on the advocate's tissue as equivalent to those of the recipient. Each cell has a twofold course of action of 6 noteworthy tissue antigens, and all of the antigens exist, in different individuals, in as much as 20 assortments. The chance of 2 people having unclear transplant antigens is around 1 of each 100,000.

An ensuing way is to calm the recipient's safe framework. This should be conceivable with earth-shattering immunosuppressive meds, for instance, cyclosporine An, or by using research focus created antibodies that assault create T cells.

Bone Marrow Transplants

When the safe response is genuinely disheartened—in babies carried into the world with invulnerable disarranges or in people with malignant growth—one potential fix is a trade of solid bone marrow. Brought into the spread, transplanted bone marrow cells can shape into working B and T cells. In bone marrow transplants, a close-by coordinate is basic. Not only is there a hazard that the body will excuse the transplanted bone marrow cells, be that as it may, create T cells from the bone marrow transplant may counterattack and obliterate the recipient's tissues. To thwart this situation, known as join versus-have sickness, analysts use meds or antibodies to "scour" the giver marrow of possibly hazardous create T cells.

Insusceptibility and Cancer

Typical cells transform into cancer cells, a portion of the antigens on their surface might change. If that the immune system sees the outside antigens, it dispatches the body's immune defenses, including killer T cells, macrophages, and NK cells. In any case, the immune system can't watch wherever to give body-wide reconnaissance, flushing out and wiping out all cells that become dangerous. Tumors develop when the system separates or is overpowered.

Researchers are forming immune cells and substances into astute new anti-cancer weapons. They are utilizing substances known as organic reaction modifiers, including lymphocytes and lymphocytes, to reinforce the patient's immune reactions. Sometimes, natural reaction modifiers are infused straightforwardly into the patient. Likewise, they can be utilized in the research facility to change a portion of the patient's lymphocytes into the hunger for tumor cells, which are then infused once again into the patient so they can attack the cancer cells.

Antibodies uniquely made to perceive explicit diseases can be combined with medications, poisons, or radioactive materials, at that point sent off like "magic bullets" to convey their deadly freight legitimately to the objective cancer cell. On the other hand, poisons can be connected to lymphocyte and directed to cells outfitted with receptors for the lymphocyte.

Radioactively labeled antibodies can likewise be utilized to find shrouded homes of cancer cells (metastases).

Still, different researchers are trying to restorative cancer vaccines; these contrast from conventional vaccines, which are given before disease beginning to shield an individual from future Infections. Cancer antibodies are utilized after the disease has emerged, and are intended to enable the immune system to fend off the disease.

The immune system regularly reacts pitifully or not in the slightest degree to cancer cells. Cancer antibodies attempt to enhance the normal anticancer reaction by animating healthy killer T-cell reactions against a tumor.

Although such antibodies are commonly not ready to annihilate a tumor whenever given as the main type of treatment, inquire about recommends they can be compelling accomplices whenever managed alongside different types of treatment.

THE IMMUNE SYSTEM AND THE NERVOUS SYSTEM

The proof is mounting that the immune system and the nervous system are connected in a few different ways. One notable association includes adrenal organs. In light of pressure messages from the brain, the adrenal organs discharge hormones into the blood. Notwithstanding helping an individual react to crises by preparing the body's vitality saves, these "stress hormones" can smother the defensive impacts of antibodies and lymphocytes.

Hormones and different chemicals are known to pass on messages among nerve cells that have been found to "talk" to cells of the immune system. Some immune cells can manufacture commonplace nerve cell items, while a few lymphocytes can transmit data to the sensory system. Also, the mind may send messages legitimately down nerve cells to the immune system. Systems of nerve strands have been found associating with the lymphoid organs.

Frontiers in Immunology

Specialists are by and by prepared to mass-produce insusceptible cell releases, the two antibodies, and lymphocytes, similarly as explicit invulnerable cells. The readied deftly of these materials not simply has changed the investigation of the invulnerable framework itself, yet furthermore has massively influenced medicine, cultivating, and industry.

Monoclonal antibodies are indistinct antibodies made by the numerous family members (clones) of a single B cell. Because of their uncommon expresses for different atoms, monoclonal antibodies are promising meds for an extent of ailments.

Specialists make monoclonal antibodies by mixing a mouse with a target antigen and a short time later interweaving B cells from the mouse with another apparently ceaseless cell. The crossover cell transforms into a type of safe reaction preparing plant, turning out vague copies of immunizer particles unequivocal for the goal antigen.

Mouse antibodies are "remote" to people, regardless, and may trigger their insusceptible reaction when mixed into a human. Thus, masters have begun to mull over "refined" monoclonal antibodies. To build up these atoms, analysts take the antigen-confining piece of a mouse immune response and affix it to a human neutralizer framework, colossally hurting the remote section of the particle.

Since they see very certain particles, monoclonal antibodies are utilized in interesting tests to perceive attacking pathogens or changes in the body's proteins. In medicate, monoclonal antibodies can append to disorder cells, obstructing the creation improvement hails that cause the cells to section crazy. In different cases, monoclonal antibodies can pass on astonishing poisons into select cells, killing the cells while leaving its neighbors faultless.

Genetic Engineering

Genetic engineering permits researchers to cull qualities—fragments of the genetic material, DNA—from one sort of organism, and join them with qualities of a subsequent life form. Along these lines, moderately basic living beings, for example, microscopic organisms or yeast, can be prompted to make amounts of human proteins, including hormones, insulin just as lymphocytes and monoclines. They can likewise produce proteins from irresistible operators, for example, the hepatitis infection or HIV, for use in vaccines.

Gene Therapy

Genetic engineering likewise holds a guarantee for quality treatment—supplanting modified or missing qualities or including supportive qualities. Extreme joined immunodeficiency illness is a prime possibility for quality treatment. SCID is brought about by the absence of a chemical because of a solitary missing quality. A hereditarily engineered rendition of the missing quality can be brought into cells taken from the patient's bone marrow. After treated marrow cells start to deliver the protein, they can be infused over into the patient.

Cancer is another objective for quality treatment. In spearheading tests, researchers are removing cancer battling lymphocytes from the disease patient's tumor, inserting a quality that helps the lymphocytes' capacity to make amounts of a characteristic anticancer item, at that point developing the rebuilt cells in an amount in the lab.

These cells are infused once again into the patient, where they can search out the tumor and convey enormous portions of the anticancer chemicals.

Immunoregulation

Research into the sensitive governing rules that control the immune reaction is expanding information on typical and unusual immune capacities. Sometimes, it might be conceivable to treat diseases, for example, fundamental lupus erythematous by stifling overly active pieces of the immune system.

Analysts have gotten by the model of the human invulnerable system by transplanting immature human resistant tissues or insusceptible cells into SCID mice. This animal model pledges to be colossally significant in helping specialists appreciate the immune system and control its bit of leeway human wellbeing.

Researchers have found out much about the immune system. They keep concentrating on how the body dispatches attacks that obliterate attacking microorganisms, tainted cells, and tumors while disregarding sound tissues. New technologies for distinguishing singular immune cells are letting researchers rapidly figure out which targets set off an immune reaction. Upgrades in microscopy are allowing the first-since forever perceptions of B cells, T cells, and different cells as they associate inside lymph nodes and other body tissues.

Furthermore, researchers are quickly unraveling the Genetic outlines that immediate the human immune reaction just as those that direct the science of microscopic organisms, parasites and infections. The mix of innovation and extended Genetic information will no uncertainty show us significantly more how the body shields itself from the disease.

Glossary

- AIDS (AIDS)— a threatening disease brought about by the human immunodeficiency infection, which separates the body's resistant guards.

- Adrenal organ—an organ situated on every kidney that secretes hormones controlling digestion, sexual capacity, water equalization, and stress.

- Allergen—any substance that causes a sensitivity, hypersensitivity—an unsafe reaction of the invulnerable system to regularly innocuous substances.

- Antibodies—particles (also called immunoglobulin) created by a B cell in light of an antigen. At the point when an immunizer connects to an antigen, it enables the body to devastate or inactivate the antigen.

- Antigen—a substance or particle that is perceived by the safe system. The particle can be from remote material, for example, microorganisms or infections.

- Antiserum—a serum wealthy in antibodies against a specific microorganism.

- Appendix—lymphoid organ in the digestive tract.

- Autoantibodies—antibodies that respond against an individual's tissue.

- Autoimmune infection—a disease that outcomes when the immune system erroneously assaults the body's tissues. Models incorporate various sclerosis, type I diabetes, rheumatoid joint inflammation, and foundational lupus erythematous.

- B cells—little white platelets urgent to the safety protections. Likewise, know as

- B lymphocytes, they originate from bone marrow and form into platelets called plasma cells, which are the wellspring of antibodies.

- Bacteria—minute creatures made out of a solitary cell. Some reason malady.

- Basophils—white platelets that add to fiery responses.

23

- Along with pole cells, basophils are answerable for the indications of hypersensitivity.
- Biological reaction modifiers—substances, either characteristic or incorporated, that help, direct, or reestablish ordinary safe barriers. They incorporate interferons, interleukins, thymus hormones, and monoclonal antibodies.
- Blood vessels—supply routes, veins, and vessels that convey blood to and from the heart and body tissues.
- Bone marrow—delicate tissue situated in the holes of the bones. Bone marrow is the wellspring of all platelets.
- Chemokine—certain proteins that animate both explicit and general invulnerable cells and help arrange resistant reactions and aggravation.
- Clone—a meeting of hereditarily indistinguishable cells or living beings slid from a solitary basic progenitor; or, imitating indistinguishable duplicates.
- Complement—a mind-boggling arrangement of blood proteins whose activity "supplements" crafted by antibodies. Supplement annihilates microorganisms, produces aggravation, and directs resistant responses.
- Complement course—an exact grouping of occasions, for the most part, activated by antigen-counter acting agent buildings, in which every segment of the supplement system is enacted thusly.
- Cytokines—incredible concoction substances emitted by cells that empower the body's cells to speak with each other.
- Cytokines incorporate lymphocytes delivered by lymphocytes and monoclines created by monocytes and macrophages.
- Cytotoxic T lymphocytes (CTLs)— a subset of T cells that convey the CD8 marker and can pulverize body cells tainted by infections or changed by malignant growth.
- DNA (deoxyribonucleic corrosive)— a long atom found in the cell core; it conveys the cell's hereditary data.

- Enzyme—a protein created by living cells that advances the synthetic procedures of existence without itself being changed.
- Eosinophil—white platelets containing granules loaded with synthetics that harm the parasites, and chemicals that influence fiery responses.
- Epithelial cells—cells making up the epithelium, the covering for inner and outer body surfaces.
- Fungi—individuals from a class of moderately crude vegetable life forms. They incorporate mushrooms, yeasts, rusts, shapes, and mucks.
- Genes—units of hereditary material (DNA) acquired from a parent. Qualities convey the directions a cell uses to play out a particular capacity.
- Graft dismissal—an invulnerable reaction against transplanted tissue.
- Graft-versus-have disease (GVHD)—a threatening response where transplanted cells assault the tissues of the beneficiary.
- Granules—layer bound organelles inside cells where proteins are put away before discharge.
- Granulocytes—phagocytic white platelets loaded up with granules life forms.
- Neutrophils, eosinophil, basophils, and pole cells are instances of granulocytes.
- Growth factors—synthetic concoctions discharged by cells that invigorate expansion of or changes in the physical properties of different cells.
- helper T cells (Th cells)— a subset of T cells that convey the CD4 surface marker and are basic for turning on counter-acting agent creation, enacting cytotoxic T cells, and starting numerous other invulnerable capacities.
- HIV (human immunodeficiency infection)—the infection that causes AIDS.

- Immune reaction—the response of the immune system to remote substances.
- Immunoglobulin—a group of enormous protein atoms, otherwise called antibodies, delivered by B cells.
- Immunosuppressive—equipped for decreasing invulnerable reactions.
- Inflammatory reaction—redness, warmth, and growing created in light of disease as the consequence of expanded bloodstream and inundation of resistant cells and discharges.
- Interferon—proteins delivered by cells that invigorate hostile to infection safe reactions or adjust the physical properties of safe cells.
- Interleukins—a significant meeting of lymphocytes and monoclines. Leukocytes—all-white platelets.
- Lymph—a straightforward, somewhat yellow liquid that conveys lymphocytes, washes the body tissues, and depletes into the lymphatic vessels.
- Lymph hubs—little bean-formed organs of the invulnerable system, dispersed broadly all through the body and connected by lymphatic vessels. Lymph hubs are battalions of B, T, and other safe cells.
- Lymphatic vessels—a body-wide system of channels, like the veins, which transport lymph to the insusceptible organs and into the circulatory system.
- Lymphocytes—little white platelets created in the lymphoid organs and central in the resistant barriers.

CHAPTER Two
"WE ARE WHAT WE EAT"

THE BEST FOOD TO BOOST IMMUNITY WITH NUTRITIONAL INFORMATION

The medical experience and countless studies conducted over decades have shown how many diseases are linked to specific nutritional deficits and can be prevented and cured by simply replenishing the deficient micronutrient in good time. Eating healthy foods can help strengthen the immune system and prevent disease and illness. Maintaining a diet rich in immunity destroyers can be more beneficial to the health of many supplements.

In order to ensure that every day you get an adequate supply of all the necessary compounds for the immune system, it is important to choose, often varying, and take the right food in the right quantities (that is, neither too much nor too little) taking into account also some important aspects of preparation and storage aimed at preserving as much as possible the nutritional value of different foods.

LEGUMES

Most legumes contain minerals, magnesium, zinc, and iron. The leguminous plant is often called "poor meat" because it is an excellent source of protein without excess saturated fat. The soluble fiber in legumes also prevents constipation and can even stabilize blood sugar. In particular:

- ### *WHOLE BEANS*
    Whole varieties contain more antioxidants, vitamins, and minerals than the refined variety. Whole grains also contain fiber that helps with proper digestion. It can help regulate bowel movements and prevent inflammation in the intestine. Whole grains also reduce C-reactive protein

levels in the body, reducing the risk of heart disease and diabetes.

VEGETABLES:

- ## BROCCOLI
  Broccoli contains sulforaphane that activates antioxidant genes and enzymes in immune cells to obtain free radicals. Broccoli can also help reverse the damage caused by oxidative stress on cells.

- ## CARROTS
  Carrots contain vitamins and minerals necessary for proper immune function. Carrots are a rich source of vitamin A that can keep cells healthy. Vitamin A also helps in the production of white blood cells, which is essential for destroying infections. More importantly, vitamin A regulates the release of immune cells into the intestine. Carrots also contain vitamins C and B, which support immune function by providing antioxidants.

- ## POTATOES
  Potatoes are rich in powerful antioxidants that can fight free radicals. It is also rich in beta carotene, which can increase T cells in the body. These T cells help immune cells fight infections. Beta carotene can also inhibit the formation of cancer cells.

- ## SQUASH
  Pumpkin provides a wide range of vitamins, minerals, and antioxidants with low calories. Pumpkin contains 145% of the required daily value of beta carotene, which is then converted into vitamin A. Vitamin A keeps the mucous membrane in the nose and mouth resistant to infections. It also contains vitamin C, which can fight most respiratory infections.

- ## TOMATOES

Tomatoes are rich in lycopene. It is a powerful antioxidant that preventscancers, including breast, pancreatic, and intestinal cancers. Studies show that organic tomatoes contain more lycopene, eaten raw, or smoothies. Tomatoes plants also contain vitamins A, C, and B6, useful for cardiovascular health. Tomatoes are also high in fiber and low in calories, so adding them to your diet is fantastic.

THE BOTANICAL FAMILY:

Onion, leek, shallot: a worthy family of vegetables. They cost a few tears, but protect against cancer, heart disease, aging... sometimes crying doesn't hurt that much. Indeed, when we talk about the Liliaceae family, the opposite is true. This is, in fact, a strange botanical family. It includes garlic, onion, shallot, leek, and chives (and even asparagus!) and is characterized, in its chemical composition, by substances that contain sulfur, which give the characteristic pungent odor. In particular:

- ## GARLIC

  Garlic is almost always included in the recipes. Not only does it add flavor to the dish, but it is also good for the immune system. A clove of garlic contains more than 100 sulfuric compounds that can kill bacteria and infections in the body. Try to consume raw garlic as heat can inactivate sulfur enzymes and reduce their antibiotic effects.

FRUITS:

- ## APPLES

  Apples contain soluble fiber, which can reduce inflammation in the body and help strengthen the immune system. Studies show that people who have eaten apples regularly are less prone to disease and have a faster recovery rate than people who have not eaten apples. Apples also contain antioxidants that strengthen the immune system and protect the body from stress.

- ## *CITRUS FRUIT*
    Citrus fruits family are rich in vitamin C, which can help the immune system to function correctly. Vitamin C is also essential in the production of collagen, which keeps the skin elastic and firm. Citrus fruits also contain flavonoids which can attack immune dysfunctions that cause cancer and inflammation.

    Eating dark green leaves can improve your overall immune function. Green leafy vegetables can activate the immune genes in the body, while processed foods can suppress it. Dark green leaves are also essential for maintaining tolerance and immunity, and reducing inflammation in the body.

- ## *FIGS AND DATES*
    Figs are rich in antioxidants, potassium, and manganese, which can regulate the body's correct pH levels. This makes it difficult for pathogens to enter the system. It can also help diabetes people with lower blood sugar levels. Dates are excellent sources of minerals and vitamins. It can prevent the growth of harmful bacteria in the intestine while stimulating the production of good bacteria in the gut.

- ## *BERRIES*
    Studies show that berries, especially Goji berries, blackberries, black currants, and blueberries, have an anti-aging effect on the immune system. Berries can also reduce inflammation and reduce stress on the body. Berries contain vitamin C and bioflavonoids, which function as antioxidants that can prevent cell damage.

Most people cannot eat 7 to 9 servings of fruit and vegetables every day. The solution is:

- ## *GREEN FOOD POWDERS*
    The green edible powder contains the necessary antioxidants and phytonutrients that can help increase immunity. Green food powders are perfect for people who

can't regularly find a new source of fruit and vegetables and for people who have an intense schedule and don't have enough time to prepare meals.

FLAX SEED

Flax seeds are one of the smallest seeds you can find in a health food store, but it has many health benefits. Flax seeds contain lignans that have anticancer properties. Flaxseeds also contain omega-three fatty acids, which can strengthen immune cells.

OATS

Oatmeal is often eaten for breakfast. Oat is very versatile and can be mixed with other ingredients such as fruit. Oatmeal contains beta-glucan, which can improve the body's ability to respond to bacterial infections. Beta-glucan can help neutrophils, a non-specific immune cell, which navigates the body. It also helps kill bacteria. Studies also show that beta-glucan in oats helps immune cells to quickly and easily locate bacteria, resulting in a rapid response to microbial infection.

OLIVE AND OLIVE OIL

Studies show that consuming olive oil can strengthen the immune system and help prevent attacks from bacteria, microorganisms, and viruses. Fatty acid in olive oil can lower immunological parameters. The fatty acids in olive oil also prevent chronic inflammation and can be used to treat autoimmune diseases.

HERBS AND SPICES

Herbs and spices are an excellent source of flavor to your dishes. But most also have therapeutic and medicinal benefits. Some herbs and spices commonly used to boost immunity are discussed below:
- Echinacea is an herb used to increase immunity. It is particularly useful in treating upper respiratory tract infections.

- Ginseng. It has anti-cancer and anti-inflammatory properties.
- Turmeric. Turmeric has antibacterial and anti-inflammatory properties. It also protects the stomach from toxins and alcohol.
- Pepper. Pepper helps correct digestion. It also reduces inflammation.
- Curry. Curry has powerful antioxidant benefits and can help prevent cell damage.
- Oregano. Oregano has active compounds called thymol and carvacrol, which have antiviral and antibacterial properties. It also helps eliminate intestinal parasites.
- Oregano. Oregano has active compounds called thymol and carvacrol, which have antiviral and antibacterial properties. It also helps eliminate intestinal parasites.

SEA VEGETABLES

Sea vegetables are one of the best foods that can help protect the body from environmental pollutants and radiation. Sea vegetables can prevent the assimilation of heavy metals and toxins. See-weed, see-weed, and see-weed are an excellent source of minerals such as potassium, iodine, and iron. Compared to vegetables grown on land, sea vegetables have higher levels of amino acids, vitamins, and minerals.

SOY FOOD

Soybeans contain flavonoids which can increase immunity against tumors. Soy-based foods are rich in antioxidants that can protect the body from free radicals. Soy products like miso also contain probiotics that maintain the right balance in the intestine and promote proper digestion. It can also reduce the risk of cancer and help lower cholesterol in the body.

NUTS AND SEEDS

Another immune system booster is the Nuts and seeds. They are an excellent source of vitamins. Almonds, hazelnuts, walnuts, and pistachios are rich in vitamin E, increasing the immunity of the elderly. It also counteracts free radicals in the body. Pumpkin seeds and sesame seeds contain zinc, which helps stabilize the immune system by increasing the number of T cells in the body. Brazilian almonds, walnuts, and walnuts have selenium, which is essential for the immune system.

YOGURT

Like any other dairy product, yogurt is also rich in calcium, vitamin B-12, and magnesium. It is also rich in probiotics or good bacteria that can help maintain the correct digestive system. Studies show that probiotics can help strengthen immunity and promote a healthier digestive system. Studies also suggest that yogurt can help people recover from an infection. Yogurt also helps prevent vaginal yeast or candida infection, which is a common problem for diabetic women.

MUSHROOMS

Mushrooms are very good foods for the immune system. Different varieties of mushrooms have various advantages. Shiitake mushrooms are said to have anti-cancer properties. Reishi mushrooms have been used for over 4,000 years because of their anti-inflammatory and antiviral properties. Maitake mushrooms resemble feathers on a chicken's tail. It is often used in immunotherapy to strengthen the immune system during radiation therapy or even chemotherapy.

A focus on the antioxidant power...

here below a list of antioxidant foods: CURCUMA, CARROTS, GREEN TEA, AVOCADO, BLACKBERRIES, MAQUI, GOJI BERRIES, RED FRUITS, KIWI and PAPAYA.

CHAPTER THREE
TASTY IMMUNE RECIPES

These are attempting times, and we need to avoid potential risk and stay at home. We additionally need to eat healthy food, nutritious, and beneficial for the immune system.

As a family, we need good dieting habits. In any case, we want to proceed and cut down on junk or carbonated beverages and prepared food (which we have every so often). It is self-restraint and limitation.

In crucial times, it is needful to have food that your body needs. You can settle on a choice to move into smart dieting habits and decisions.

I am sharing vegeterian-lover plant-based recipes and food, which I prepared at home. I won't get over the edge as an abundance of every single thing isn't acceptable. Balance is key. But, I might want to incorporate a greater amount of these immune-boosting foods in our eating diets than prior.

Note: If you have allergies to specific nourishments or an uncommon disease, then generously counsel your primary care physician. For example, Papaya isn't acceptable during pregnancy. Wheatgrass is likewise superb for boosting the immune system; however, it won't suit everyone and may hurt. So remember your body condition and constitution.

Immune Boosting Vegetarian Foods

Natural products: Oranges, Pomegranate, Apple, Sweet Limes, Guava, Fresh Berries, Tomato, Amla (Indian Gooseberry), Lemon.

Vegetables:, Carrots, Broccoli, Sweet Potato, Eggplant (Brinjal), Bell Pepper (Capsicum), Spinach, Cabbage, Beets, Moringa, Dill Leaves (Suva).

Nuts and Seeds: Almonds (splashed for the time being), Walnuts, Fennel Seeds, Sunflower seeds.

Herbs, Roots, Spices: Ginger, Turmeric, Garlic, Giloy (Guduchi), Basil, Ashwagandha, Tulsi (Holy Basil).

Beverages: Coconut water, Green tea, freshly arranged fruit juices plentiful in Vitamin C. Dodge carbonated sweet beverages, liquor, and handled nourishments. Have a lot of water.

Probiotic Foods: Buttermilk, Sauerkraut, Kefir, Kimchi, Curd or Yogurt (with live and dynamic societies), Carrot Kanji ,Kombucha.

Important healthy advances

1. Kindly limit the use of refined sugar in these recipes. Any place conceivable supplants sugar with better choices like jaggery, maple syrup, grungy sugar, coconut sugar, agave syrup. You can likewise utilize nectar however, don't warm it.

2. Avoid including ice cubes to drinks and avoid utilizing cold water to make those beverages. Summer is drawing closer, and we as a whole prefer to have cold beverages during summers. But, drinking warm water (with cumin seeds) or hot beverages is going to help.

3. Salted lukewarm or lukewarm turmeric water rinsing is additionally going to help.

4. Don't indulge and ensure you can process the food. Bite food well and eat it in a happy environment.

5. Lastly, get adequate rest, do direct yoga or exercise, practice meditation, don't frenzy, and remain loose. All of these means like having deep, peaceful sleep, doing direct yoga, practicing meditation or body-mind loosening up strategies, praying, tuning in to alleviating music, or viewing a parody film or religious show will likewise assist you with building immunity.

6. Happiness, inspiration, laughter, loosened up mind are few feelings that will give you a healthy, passionate, and mental prosperity. So center on positivity, trust, love, and healing. Spread the vibrations of love, energy, and harmony. Recollect this also will pass if we are as one in our purpose to battle but then detached at our home. Remain Immune, Stay at home, Stay Healthy, and also Be Positive.

Immune Boosting Drinks

Healthy Strawberry Smoothie

This strawberry smoothie is a rich, delightful smoothie full-on with the taste and flavors of strawberries —Sans gluten and vegetarian.

To thicken the smoothie, I utilized one banana, yet it very well may be effortlessly skipped.

Ingredients

- 200 grams of strawberries - cleaved and hulled or 1.25 cups of chopped strawberries
- ½ cup coconut milk - slender to medium consistency
- 1 medium-huge banana

Instructions

1. Wash hull and afterward chop strawberries. Include them in a mixer or mixer.
2. Add 1 medium to huge banana (chopped).
3. Pour ½ cup of coconut milk having a medium or thin consistency. You can include some sugar like maple syrup, coconut sugar, or nectar if you need it. For thick smoothie, you can add ¼ to ⅓ cup of coconut milk.
4. Mix till smooth.
5. Pour into glasses and serve strawberry smoothie.

Notes

- This recipe can be significantly increased.
- You can include sugar of your decision.
- You can likewise utilize cow's milk rather than coconut milk.

Turmeric Tea

Turmeric tea is a healthy and recuperating drink. I make the tea myself.

I have turmeric tea at night time or now and again before hitting the bed. It revives me as well as causes me to feel better.

Advantages of Turmeric and Other Spices

Turmeric – Curcumin in turmeric has amazing cancer antioxidant agents and anti-inflammatory properties. It helps immunity and useful for the skin as well. You can include either new turmeric roots or ground turmeric powder in the recipe.

Black Pepper –anti-inflammatory and Antioxidant properties can also be found in black pepper. Likewise, black pepper assists in engrossing curcumin. It additionally invigorates hunger and aids indigestion.

Ceylon Cinnamon – Aromatic Ceylon cinnamon has anti-inflammatory, antioxidant, and antimicrobial properties. It is additionally useful for immunity. Generously note to utilize genuine cinnamon or Ceylon cinnamon in any recipe and not cassia cinnamon.

Ginger –ginger roots contain gingerol, which has antioxidant benefits. Ginger additionally helps in digestion, harmful nausea and helps in soothing chop and cold. In the recipe, you can utilize both new ground ginger or ginger root powder.

Instructions to Make Turmeric Tea

1. In a pot, take 1 cup of water. Water in a pan

2. Add ½ to 1 tablespoon of raw, grungy sugar. You can even utilize jaggery or maple syrup or skirt the sugar. Including grungy raw sugar

3. Let the water reach a boiling point and include ⅛ teaspoon ground ginger (dried ginger powder – saunth). ½ teaspoon of newly ground ginger root or squashed ginger can likewise be included. Including dry ginger powder when the water reaches boiling point

4. Next include ⅛ teaspoon of ground Ceylon cinnamon (Ceylon cinnamon powder and not cassia cinnamon powder) including ground Ceylon cinnamon powder

5. Include ⅛ teaspoon of squashed black pepper or ground black pepper. Including squashed black pepper

6. Include ½ teaspoon of ground (turmeric powder). adding ground turmeric powder

7. Bubble further for a moment or two turmeric tea boiling

37

8. Expel pan and pour the tea in a mug. You can also strain the tea while pouring. Appreciate turmeric tea hot.

IMMUNE BOOSTING SOUPS

Palak Soup | Spinach Soup

The Palak soup recipe. Here is one simple and delicious low-calorie Spinach soup recipe. I love soups and particularly when it's coming down or during wintertime. It is too ameliorating even to consider sipping and taste from a bowl of steaming sweltering soup in a chilly climate.

Ingredients

- 1.5 to 2 cups spinach (palak), chopped
- ¼ cup onions, chopped
- 2 to 3 garlic cloves, finely chopped
- 1 tablespoon gram flour (besan)
- ¼ teaspoon cumin powder
- 1 tejpatta (Indian narrows leaf) - little size
- 2 cups of water
- 1 or 1.5 tablespoon olive oil or margarine
- Black pepper powder as required
- Salt as required
- Cream for ingredients (discretionary)
- Some newly squashed black pepper or ground cheddar or paneer/curds or cream for embellishing - discretionary

Instructions

1. First, flush the palak leaves (spinach) very well in water.
2. At that point, slash the palak leaves and keep aside.
3. sauteing and cooking spinach soup mix
4. Warmth oil or margarine in a saucepan. Include the narrows leaf and fry for 2-3 seconds
5. Presently include the chopped garlic and fry till the garlic is lightly carmelized or sautéed. Try not to consume garlic.

6. Saute the garlic on a low fire. Include chopped onions and saute till the onions are relaxed.

7. Include the chopped palak/spinach. Mix and season with black pepper and salt.

8. Presently include the besan or gram flour. Mix well and pour 2 cups water.

9. Heat the mix to the point of boiling and afterward stew for 3-4 minutes.

10. Include cumin powder and mix well.

11. Switch off the fire and let the soup mixture cool.

12. making spinach soup

13. At the point when the mix's warmth has decreased or has gotten warm, at that point mix with a hand mixer or in a mixer till smooth.

14. Evacuate the tejpatta (Indian straight leaf) while mixing.

15. Check the flavoring and include some increasingly salt or pepper whenever required.

16. If the soup looks thick, at that point, include 1/4 or 1/2 cup water and mix.

17. Hold the very much mixed soup back on the oven for stewing for 2-3 minutes.

18. Serve spinach soup hot sprinkled with some newly squashed black pepper or ground paneer, cheddar or beat with some cream.

Carrot Soup (One Pot)

Carrot soup is made simple with a recipe that gives you a delicious one pot, a thick and rich soup that you will make over and over again. The recipe is likewise vegetarian and without gluten.

Ingredients

- 400 grams of carrots or 0.9 pounds of carrots or 2.25 cups chopped carrots or 8 to 10 small to medium-sized carrots - diced or cubed

- 2 tablespoons of chopped celery

- ¼ to ½ teaspoon freshly squashed black pepper
- 1 to 2 teaspoons of chopped cilantro (coriander leaves)
- ¼ teaspoon of lemon juice - discretionary
- ½ teaspoon cumin seeds
- ½ teaspoon salt or include according to taste
- 1 tablespoon of oil - sunflower or additional virgin olive oil. margarine can likewise be subbed
- ½ cup chopped onions or 1 medium-sized onion or 60 grams onion
- ½ teaspoon chopped garlic or 2 to 3 little to medium-sized garlic cloves
- 2.5 cups vegetable stock or water
- ¼ to ½ cup water - while mixing, discretionary

For garnish
- 1 teaspoon chopped cilantro or chopped parsley (coriander leaves)
- ⅓ cup of bread garnishes - discretionary

Guidelines
1. In a thick bottomed pan, olive oil or sunflower on a low to medium-low fire. Include chopped garlic and onions.
2. Sauté on a low to medium-low fire till the onions can relax.
3. Include chopped carrots, celery, cumin seeds, and salt. Mix well.
4. Pour 2.5 cups vegetable stock or water. Mix and mix once more.
5. Spread pot with a top. Stew on a low or medium-low fire till the carrots become delicate.
6. When stewing, do check a few times to check whether the fluids have dried or not. If the fluids have dried, add ¼ to ½ cup a greater amount of hot veg stock or high temp water.

7. Check a couple of bits of carrots with a fork or blade. The fork or blade ought to have the option to pass effectively from the carrots.

8. After the carrots are cooked, switch off the fire. There will be some fluid in the mix. Let this fluid stay as we will utilize these fluids when mixing the carrots. Let the soup mix become warm or less hot.

Making carrot soup

1. Include the whole mix with the fluids in a mixer or processor. You can even utilize a drenching mixer to mix the carrots.

2. Mix to a smooth puree. While mixing, add ¼ to ½ cup of water (at room temperature) depending upon the thickness you incline toward in the soup.

3. Place the whole pureed carrots in a similar pot.

4. Keep the pan on burner and stew till the soup gets really hot. Mix at interims. If the carrot soup looks thick, at that point, you can include some increasingly high temp water.

5. At the point when the soup gets hot, season with chopped parsley and black pepper; mix well, then switch off the fire. Rather than parsley, you can even utilize new cilantro. This is a discretionary advance. For some blackout sharp notes in the soup, you can include ¼ teaspoon of lemon juice.

6. serving carrot soup

7. Serve carrot soup in mugs. Embellishment with some cilantro or parsley. Add some bread garnishes if you like.

8. Bread garnishes truly taste great in this soup. To make bread garnishes simply toast a 1 or maybe 2-day old bread or roll in the broiler or on a pan (Tawa). At the point when toasted, cut them in small cubes and present with carrot soup.

Notes

- Making carrot soup in the moment pot:

- Utilize the sauté choice and sauté onions, garlic typical till the onions mollify.
- Press drop. At that point include carrots, salt, celery and cumin. Mix well.
- Include 2 cups of vegetable stock or water.
- Close with top and place the valve in the ingredients position.
- Press the weight cook catch and weight cook for 10 minutes.
- Sit tight for 5 minutes. At that point following 5 minutes do a snappy weight discharge by carrying the valve.
- Let the mix chill off a piece and afterward mix in a mixer or utilizing an inundation mixer to a smooth puree.
- From the mixer, pour the carrots in the moment pot steel embed.
- If the puree looks really thick, include some heated water.
- Press the drop button. At that point, press the catch and set time to 2 minutes on ordinary. Let the soup become warm or hot. Mix at interims.
- Include parsley and black pepper. Mix and serve.

Some more tips:
- Both orange and red carrots can be utilized in the recipe.
- Use carrots that are new and delicate. Stay away from carrots, which are stringy and hard.
- Water can be included rather than vegetable stock.
- Best to use handcrafted vegetable stock and not the canned ones because of the high sodium content.
- Any nonpartisan enhanced oil can be utilized. You can even utilize margarine to make a veggie-lover carrot soup.
- You can include seasonings, flavors of your decision in the carrot soup. Yet, do remember the taste and flavor of carrots with the aim that the seasonings or flavors bring out the best as far as taste and flavor in the soup.

- Extra carrot soup could be refrigerated and afterward heated up before serving. If the soup turns out to be thick, at that point, include some water and warm it.

SIDE DISHES FOR GOOD IMMUNITY

Yam Chaat Recipe

Yam chaat is one of the least demanding to plan chaat recipe with yams or shakarkandi.

Ingredients

- 260 to 270 grams yams or 1.5 to 2 cups chopped bubbled yams (shakarkandi)
- ¼ teaspoon black pepper powder (kali Mirch powder)
- ½ teaspoon amchur powder (dry mango powder) or include as required
- ½ to 1 teaspoon lemon juice
- rock salt or sendhanamak as required

Instructions

1. Right off the bat, wash 260 to 270 yams very well in water.
2. At that point, steam them in a weight cooker or a dish. If cooking in a weight cooker, at that point, pressure cook for around 3 to 4 whistles with water pretty much covering the yams.

Making shakarkandikichaat:

1. After the yams are cooked well and when they become warm, at that point, pill them gently and slash them. Take them in a bowl.
2. Include 1/4 teaspoon black pepper powder, 1/2 teaspoon amchur powder (dry mango powder) and rock salt (sendhanamak). If making for customary days, at that point, you can likewise include red bean stew powder and chaat masala powder. Some cooked cumin powder can likewise be included. You can include the zest powders less or more according to your taste inclinations.
3. At that point 1/2 to 1 teaspoon lemon juice.

4. Mix tenderly. Check the taste and include any of the flavor powders or lemon juice whenever required.

5. Serve shakarkandi ki chaat.

Notes

Tips for making shakarkandi ki chaat recipe:

- You can likewise include 1/4 to 1/2 teaspoon cooked cumin powder in the recipe.
- The recipe can be effectively multiplied or significantly increased.
- If not making for Navratri fasting, at that point, you can utilize red bean stew powder, chaat masala.
- Black salt can likewise be included rather than rock salt.
- Flavor powders can be included pretty much according to your taste inclinations.

Amla Pickle | Indian Gooseberry Pickle

This vegetarian amla pickle is Andhra style hot and scrumptious pickle made with Indian gooseberry, flavors, lemon juice, and oil.

Ingredients

- 250 grams amla or around 2 cups chopped amla (Indian gooseberry)
- ⅓ cup sesame oil (gingelly oil) for singing amla
- 2 tablespoons of mustard seeds or 3 tablespoon mustard seeds powder
- ¼ teaspoon fenugreek seeds
- 3 tablespoons of red bean stew powder
- 2 to 3 little to medium garlic cloves - marginally squashed
- 1 teaspoon of turmeric powder
- 1 to 1.5 tablespoons of salt or add as required
- ¼ cup sesame oil - to be included later
- ¼ teaspoon asafoetida (hing)
- 1 tablespoon of lemon juice

Guidelines

1. Right off the bat, rinse the amla very well with water. At that point, clean dry with a perfect kitchen towel. Or on the other hand, you can spread on a cotton napkin or on a plate and let them dry normally.

2. At that point in a processor, include 2 tablespoons of mustard seeds and ¼ teaspoon of fenugreek seeds.

3. Crush to a semi-fine powder. Keep aside.

Cooking amla

1. Chop the amla and expel the seeds. Chopping amla requires some investment. If the amla is little in size, at that point, you can keep them entirety.

2. Warmth ⅓ cup sesame oil in a Kadai or dish.

3. Include the chopped amla pieces. Mix well.

4. Spread the dish and allow the amla pieces to cook with oil in the middle of doing a check.

5. You don't have to cook the amla pieces till brilliant. They ought to be cooked until they relax. Slid a blade through a couple of pieces, and it ought to slide without any problem. This cooking on a medium-low fire takes around 6 to 7 minutes.

6. Once the amla is cooked, then switch off the fire. Add 2 to 3 medium garlic cloves (squashed). Mix well and until the mixture becomes warm. Save aside for around 5 to 10 minutes and leave the amla pieces in the container as it were.

Preparing amla pickle

1. Include 3 tablespoons of red bean stew powder, 1 to 1.5 tablespoons of salt, 1 teaspoon of turmeric powder, and the blend mustard seeds with fenugreek powder. First, include 1 tablespoon salt. Mix well indeed. If less salt, at that point, include some progressively salt. If the pickle tastes really salty, at that point, it's fine as when it develops, the extra salty taste leaves.

2. Mix well indeed. Let this mix chill off at room temperature.

3. Presently include a tablespoon lemon juice. Mix once more.

4. Place the pickle in a clean, disinfected container. Spread with a cover and keep aside treating for amla pickle

5. Presently heat cup oil in a little dish or tadka container. This progression is discretionary and can be skipped.

6. Hold fire to a low and include ¼ teaspoon asafoetida (hing).

7. Mix well and afterward switch off the fire. Let the oil cool off.

8. At that point, pour the oil into the pickling container. Some oil will spill on top, and its fine. Spread the container with a top and let the pickle develop for 3 to 4 days. Keep in a dry place.

9. Serve amla pickle with your supper. After you start to utilize the pickle, make sure to refrigerate it.

Notes
- Include less red bean stew powder for a zesty pickle.
- You can darkish the measure of oil if you need it.
- Rather than sesame oil, nut oil or sunflower oil can be utilized.

IMMUNE BOOSTING MAIN COURSE RECIPES

Kale Leaves Recipe With Mushroom | Kale, And Mushrooms In Ginger Sauce

Kale leaves recipe – kale leaves and catches mushrooms in a daintily spiced ginger sauce. I had made this kale and mushrooms in the ginger sauce as a going with a side dish with schezwan singed rice.

Ingredients
- 8 to 10 kale leaves
- 8 to 10 catch mushrooms

- 1 spring onions (scallions) - save the greens for embellishing
- 2 to 3 garlic - finely chopped
- 1 or 2 green chilies - finely chopped
- 1-inch ginger - finely chopped
- 1 teaspoon light soy sauce or as required
- ½ teaspoon sugar or as required
- ¼ teaspoon black pepper powder or as required
- 1 tablespoon bolt root flour or (corn starch + 1/3 cup water). I included bolt root flour
- 1.5 tablespoon oil
- ½ to ¾ cup water or as required
- Salt as required

Instructions

1. Wash and cut the mushrooms.
2. Wash and leave the kale leaves. You can cut off the central stem if you like. I typically keep them.
3. Warmth oil in a container. Include the ginger, garlic and green chilies and saute for a couple of moments.
4. Include the spring onions/scallions and saute for 1 or 2 minutes.
5. Include the mushrooms and pan-fried food the mushrooms on a high warmth untill the mushroom is cooked from the edges.
6. Include the chopped kale leaves. Saute till the leaves become delicate. Around 7 to 8 minutes.
7. Include soy sauce and mix well.
8. At that point, include 1/2 to 3/4 cup water and bring to a stew.
9. Break up 1 tbsp bolt root flour or corn starch in 1/3 cup water.
10. Include this mix in the dish. Stew till the sauce thickens and gets smooth with a coating.

11. Season with salt, pepper, and sugar.
12. Garnish with scallion greens and serve kale and mushrooms in ginger sauce hot with seared rice or steamed rice.

Notes

Options for kale - since kale leaves are not accessible in India. Here are not many alternatives:

1. You could include kohlrabi (ganthgobi) greens. Be that as it may, the leaves ought to be delicate and young.
2. Collard greens can likewise be included. They are known as Karamsaag and added to plan Haak, a Kashmiri dish.
3. Malabar spinach. Otherwise, called Puisaag in Bengali.
4. Indeed, even Chinese cabbage bokchoy would be acceptable. 5. You can attempt spinach as well, yet spinach won't hold its shape and nibble like kale.

Cauliflower Curry

- Cauliflower curry recipe sound and delectable cauliflower curry that goes very well with rice parathas or chapatis.
- Cauliflower curry is a sound and heavenly curry that goes very well with rice or chapatis.

Ingredients

- ½ teaspoon coriander powder
- ½ teaspoon garam masala powder
- 300 grams cauliflower or 2.5 to 3 cups slashed cauliflower
- 2 tablespoons oil
- 1 green bean stew - slashed
- ¼ teaspoon turmeric powder
- ½ teaspoon Kashmiri red bean stew powder
- ½ teaspoon cumin seeds
- 1 medium onion - finely divided, or ⅓ cup slashed onions

- 1.5 teaspoons ginger-garlic stick
- 2 medium tomatoes divided or 1 cup hacked tomatoes
- ¼ teaspoon Kasurimethi - crushed (dry fenugreek leaves)
- 2 to 3 tablespoons hacked coriander leaves
- (cilantro leaves)
- (ground coriander)
- ¾ to 1 cup water or incorporate as required
- Salt as required

Bearings

- Warmth 2 tablespoons oil in a dish or Kadai.
- Include ½ teaspoon cumin seeds and let them splutter.
- At that point, incorporate ⅓ cup cleaved onions.
- Saute the onions on medium-low fire till they become translucent.
- Next, incorporate 1.5 teaspoons ginger-garlic stick or crushed ginger-garlic.
- Mix and saute the ginger-garlic, till the crude aroma of ginger-garlic leaves.
- Diminish the fire to a low. By then, incorporate ¼ teaspoon turmeric powder, ½ teaspoon Kashmiri red stew powder, and ½ teaspoon coriander powder.
- Keep the fire low, blend the flavors very well. You can get even mood killer the fire.
- Next, incorporate 1 cup severed tomatoes and 1 green stew (slashed).
- Mix the tomatoes very well and begin to saute them on a low to medium-low fire.
- Saute till the tomatoes become smooth, getting delicate and seeing oil releasing from sides of the dish.

- At that point, add 2.5 to 3 cups cleaved cauliflower florets. You can even brighten the cauliflower in high temp water for 15 to 20 minutes if you need.
- Mix the cauliflower very well with the masala.
- Season with salt as indicated by taste. Blend well, to be sure.

Cooking cauliflower curry

- At that point, add ¾ to 1 cup water or include as required.
- Spread the compartment with a top and cook on a low to medium-low fire till the cauliflower is cooked and fragile.
- Do check-in, and if the water dissipates, you can incorporate more water.
- When the cauliflower is done, by then incorporate ¼ teaspoon Kasurimethi. Squash the Kasuri methi and a short time later incorporate it.
- Mix again well and switch off the fire.
- Ultimately, add 2 to 3 tablespoons divided coriander leaves. Blend well.
- Serve cauliflower curry with chapatis or steamed rice. You can, in like manner, serve it as a side dish with a combo of dal-rice or any veg sauce and rice.

Healthy Office Snacks to keep you Energized and Productive

Having nutritious snacks to eat during the workday can help you with staying enabled and productive.

Taking everything into account, considering musings for snacks that are difficult to prepare, healthy, and can be troublesome.

Here are fundamental and healthy snacks for work.

1. Nuts and dried fruit

Nuts and dried fruit make for a healthy, strong snack blend.

This filling combo has a decent evening out of every one of the three macronutrients, with healthy fats and protein from nuts and carbs from dried natural fruits. Moreover, the two nourishments are stacked with fiber that can help keep you full between dinners.

2. Ring peppers and guacamole

Guacamole is a scrumptious dive generally delivered utilizing avocados, lime, onion, and cilantro. It goes amazing with other raw veggies or ringer pepper.

Likewise, avocados are high in monounsaturated fats that have been seemed to help with healthy blood cholesterol levels and heart wellbeing.

3.Avocado and brown rice cake

Brown rice cakes are a stunning, rack stable snack for the work environment. Brown rice cake (19 grams) gives 14 grams of carbs and 4% of the Daily Value (DV) for fiber for only 60 calories.

Avocados are high in sound fats and fiber. Cutting or spreading the pounded fruit on a rice cake makes for a wonderful bite.

Make sure to look for rice cakes that are made with simply rice and salt and don't have futile ingredients.

4. Cooked chickpeas

Cooked chickpeas are a healthy snack that is high in protein, fiber, and a couple of supplements and minerals.

A 1/2 cup (125 grams) of chickpeas has 5 grams of fiber and 10 grams of protein. Likewise, they contain most by far of the amino acids your body might need, so their protein is seen as of higher caliber than that of various vegetables.

Research has shown that eating vegetables with great protein can help improve sentiments of completion and may help weight reduction.

To make cooked chickpeas, channel a jar of chickpeas and pat dry. Throw them in olive oil, sea salt, and seasonings of your choice and get ready on a lined warming sheet at 350°F (180°C) for 40 minutes.

5. Fish pockets

Vacuum-fixed fish pockets are useful snacks that don't should to be drained and can be taken care of and eaten at work.

Fish is stacked with filling protein and omega-3 unsaturated fats that are known to battle irritation and may lessen your risk of heart illness.

Fish pockets are commonly open in stores and on the web. Search for varieties that contain light skipjack fish, which is lower in mercury than various types.

6. Apples and nut spread

Apple cuts with typical nut spread make for a luscious, satisfying snack.

Nut spread contributes protein and healthy fats, while apples are high in fiber and water, making them particularly filling. Honestly, 1 medium apple (182 grams) is over 85% water and has various grams of fiber.

7. Jerky

Jerky is a rack consistent, high protein snack that can satisfy your craving during the workday.

One ounce (28 grams) of cheeseburger has 8 grams of protein for only 70 calories. Moreover, it's copious in iron, a huge mineral for keeping up blood wellbeing and imperativeness levels.

Quest for jerky that is uncured, low in sodium, and delivered utilizing barely any ingredients. You can, in like manner, find turkey, chicken, and salmon jerky if you don't eat red meat.

8. Carefully assembled granola

Granola spares well in your work area cabinet for a snappy bite.

As most privately procured varieties are high in included sugars and contain terrible vegetable oils that may grow your body's disturbance, it's optimal to make your own.

Simply join moved oats, sunflower seeds, cashews, dried cranberries in a blend of melted coconut oil and nectar, spread the blend out on a lined planning sheet, and warm around 40 minutes at low warmth.

This blend is healthy, balanced, and well off in complex carbs, fiber, and healthy fats. Likewise, the dissolvable fiber in oats could help lower cholesterol levels and improve heart wellbeing.

9. Greek yogurt

Plain, unsweetened Greek yogurt is a good work bite that is higher in protein than just ordinary yogurt.

A 6-ounce (170-gram) holder of plain, low-fat Greek yogurt has 17 grams of protein for only 140 calories. Additionally, it's stacked with calcium, a mineral that is critical for healthy teeth and bones.

To make this treat impressively progressively delightful and filling, incorporate healthy verdant nourishments.

10. Edamame

Edamame is young soybeans that can be enjoyed steamed, dried, or cooked.

They're stacked with first-class, plant-based protein. Without a doubt, considers shows that the protein in soy is also as satisfying as cheeseburger protein and may assist hunger with controlling and weight decrease.

11. Popcorn

Popcorn is a nutritious and satisfying snack for work that is high in fiber and low in calories. Two cups (16 grams) of air-popped popcorn give 62 calories, 2 grams of fiber, 12 grams of carbs, and a couple of supplements and minerals.

Moreover, it contains antioxidants called polyphenols that may help guarantee against constant conditions, for instance, a heart ailment.

12. Cottage cheese and fruits

Protein-rich curds and a normal item is a healthy bite that is perfect for work. It's very low in calories yet stacked with essential supplements. A 1/2 cup (113 grams) of low-fat curds has 12 grams of protein and 10% of the DV for calcium for only 80 calories.

You can bring pre-regulated servings of curds to work and top it with a natural item, for instance, cut berries, and a healthy fat source like pumpkin seeds.

13. Warmed veggie chips

Warmed or got dried out veggie chips are a healthy, rack stable bite. In any case, some privately gained varieties are made with vegetable oils, such as canola or soybean oil, and contain futile included substances.

Making your veggie chips permits you to control the ingredients you use.

Gently cut sweet potatoes, beets, carrots, zucchini, or radishes and brush them with a restricted amount of olive oil. Get ready on a lined warming sheet at 225°F (110°C) for around 2 hours.

14. Ants on a log

Ants on a log are a sound bite made with celery sticks, nut spread, and raisins. They contain sound fats, protein, and moderate devouring carbs and fiber that can give an expansion in essentialness to your workday.

Additionally, celery is for the most part water, which makes it particularly filling for a low-calorie food.

15. Homemade energy balls

Vitality balls are normally delivered utilizing oats; nut spread, sugar, and other incorporate ins like dried leafy nourishments.

Dependent upon the ingredients, they're high in fiber, sound fats, protein, and a couple of supplements and minerals.

To make your own, mix 1 cup (80 grams) of moved oats with 1/2 cup (128 grams) of nut spread, 2 tablespoons (14 grams) of ground flax seeds, 1/4 cup (85 grams) of nectar, and 1/4 cup (45 grams) of dull chocolate chips.

Fold a spoonful of the blend into diminished down balls and welcome it as a treat all through your workday.

You can discover many other vitality ball plans on the web or in particular books.

16. Cereal parcels

Keeping plain, unsweetened oat allocates by caught up with working is an unprecedented strategy to stay arranged with healthy bites.

Plain oats are high in engaging carbs and dissolvable fibers, which seemed to help lower cholesterol levels and improve heart wellbeing.

17. Carrots and hummus

Hummus is a tasty dive created utilizing chickpeas, tahini, garlic, olive oil, and lemon crush that go mind-blowing with carrots.

Hummus contains fiber, protein, and healthy fats, while carrots are stacked with beta carotene, a harbinger for a supplement in your body.

Eating nourishments with beta carotene can help bolster resistance and advance the perfect vision and eye wellbeing.

18. Dim chocolate-covered nuts

Dark chocolate-covered nuts are a nutritious, sweet treat that you can acknowledge in the working environment.

In particular, dark chocolate is rich in antioxidants that can fight particles considered free radicals that hurt cells and are associated with various interminable illnesses.

Moreover, nuts contribute protein and healthy fats that can help top you off.

Search for brands that don't contain included sugars and use dark chocolate with at any rate a large portion of full-scale cocoa content, as it has a more noteworthy amount of antioxidants than various assortments.

19. Reheat able egg rolls

Egg rolls delivered utilizing beaten eggs, cheese, and veggies are a sound, in a hurry, food.

Eggs are stacked with first-class protein and numerous supplements and minerals. To be sure, 1 egg gives over 20% of the DV for choline, a fundamental complement for your mind.

To make your egg scones get beaten raw eggs together with chopped veggies and cheese. Empty the blend into lubed roll tins and get ready at 375°F (190°C) for 15–20 minutes.

To warm an egg roll at work, place it in the microwave for 60–90 seconds or until it's warmed through.

20. Clementine and almonds

Almonds and Clementine are two healthy nourishments that you can without a lot of a stretch eat at work for a mid-night snack.

Together they give really good equality of fiber, protein, and sound fats that can help keep you full longer than a clementine alone.

Additionally, 1 clementine (74 grams) has close to 60% of the DV for supplement C, a critical supplement for healing tissue, wound recuperating, and immunity.

21. String cheese

String cheese is a profitable bite stacked with important supplements.

One string cheese (28 grams) has 80 calories, 6 grams of protein, and 15% of the DV for calcium. Eating low-calorie nourishments that are high in protein can help top you off, decrease for the most part calorie affirmation, and help weight decrease.

22. Spiced cashews

Spiced cashews make for an especially nutritious bite. They contain heart-healthy fats, similarly as supplements and minerals. Likewise, these nuts are rich in the cell fortification's lutein and zeaxanthin that are irreplaceable for suitable eye work.

In all honesty, high affirmations of lutein and zeaxanthin have been associated with a lower peril old enough related macular degeneration.

To make this flavorful treat, hurl crude cashews in olive oil, cumin, ginger and bean stew powder. Spread them on a lined, getting ready sheet and warmth in the oven at 325°F (165°C) for 12–15 minutes.

You can moreover buy spiced cashews in stores and on the internet. Basically, make sure to pick an assortment that uses irrelevant, standard ingredients.

The guide to antioxidant foods

Antioxidants are compounds that may help concede or even forestall cell harm in the body. Exactly when an individual uses them in immense totals, antioxidants may help monitor the body against oxidative concern from possibly damaging free radicals, which are unstable particles.

Exactly when free radicals create in a person's blood, they can make oxidative pressure. Oxidative pressure may extend the risk of making malignant growth, heart ailment, and many different unending infections and clinical issues.

Many stimulating nourishments contain antioxidants. If an individual eats up a couple, or these nourishments ordinarily, they may extend their cell antioxidants levels, possibly helping them forestall the damage that specialists partner with oxidative pressure.

In this book, we show likely the most refreshing nourishments that an individual can eat to help the antioxidants in their eating schedule.

1. Blueberries

Blueberries are well off in supplements while also being low in calories. An ongoing report showed that wild blueberries contain incalculable antioxidants.

Studies on blueberries have shown that these characteristic items have beneficial effects due to their antioxidant content. For example, the authors of a review of animal examine contemplated that antioxidants in blueberries may have restorative uses for neurological conditions, incorporating those that relate to developing.

A 2016 study investigated the anthocyanin that happens ordinarily in blueberries and other plant materials. Anthocyanin has a spot with a get-together of synthetics that have antioxidants and quieting exercises. They are liable for an extensive part of the splendid shades of results of the dirt.

The review found that anthocyanins may help hinder raised degrees of low thickness lipoprotein (LDL), or horrendous, cholesterol, similarly as cutting down the risk of heart ailment and diminishing a person's circulatory strain.

2. Dull chocolate

Incredible quality dull chocolate has critical degrees of supplements and cancer prevention agents. Specialists have associated dim chocolate to the extent of potential clinical favorable circumstances, including:

- the lower threat of heart disease
- decreased aggravation
- less chance of hypertension
- advancement of good cholesterol

One study of 10 sorts of research, including close to 300 individuals, demonstrated that dark chocolate reduces both upper and lower beat estimations.

The creator noted, regardless, that future research needs to choose how much dull chocolate an individual should eat for these favorable circumstances and investigate its effect on other metabolic conditions.

3. Artichokes

Artichokes give lots of supplements and cell reinforcements. The examination suggests that they may help lower with individuals' cholesterol levels and improve their gut wellbeing.

One research investigating the helpful usage of artichokes after some time saw that artichoke use could be valuable for gut, liver, and heart wellbeing.

Another exploration showed that synthetic compounds creations in artichokes had antioxidants sway on LDL cholesterol in examine focus tests. Along these lines, routinely eating up artichokes may add to cutting down a person's peril of cardiovascular infections and other related conditions.

How people plan artichokes has any sort of impact on their cell reinforcement levels. One investigation thought regarding bubbling, broiling, and steaming to see how each impacted the cell reinforcement levels.

The results showed that steaming extended the sufficiency of the cell antioxidants by various occasions while bubbling extended it eightfold. Scientists acknowledge the clarification behind this is coming and steaming separate the cell dividers, making the antioxidants levels.

4. Pecans

Pecans offer noteworthy degrees of good fat, calories, minerals, and cancer prevention agents.

One investigation showed that the body can hold cell antioxidants from pecans and grow their blood levels.

It furthermore found that eating crude pecans cuts down the blood levels of oxidized LDL cholesterol, which may suggest that these nuts help hinder heart disease.

5. Strawberries

Strawberries are copious in antioxidants, supplements, and minerals. Strawberries owe their red colors to anthocyanin, which has cell reinforcement powers.

A 2016 review showed that taking anthocyanin supplements diminished the LDL cholesterol's degrees in individuals with raised cholesterol. By cutting down LDL cholesterol levels, anthocyanin may help prevent heart sickness.

People can eat up crude strawberries as a bite or as a part of a plate of salad or different dishes.

In spite of the fact that strawberries are ingredients in some warmed product, these things are only from time to time invigorating and are not a decent choice for people endeavoring to get fit as a fiddle.

6. Red cabbage

Red cabbage contains numerous commendations, including supplements A, C, and K, notwithstanding a couple of cell reinforcements.

Red cabbage, like strawberries and red kale, contains anthocyanin. Despite giving the vegetable its red colors, this social affair of cell antioxidants progresses heart wellbeing, forestall disease, and diminishes irritation.

As demonstrated by one research, anthocyanin has the going with clinical points of interest:

- anti-combustible
- anticancer
- diabetes upkeep and the board
- promote weight control
- prevent heart sickness

In any case, more research is so far imperative to choose the wellbeing effects of eating red cabbage. An individual can eat red cabbage as a part of a serving of salad or as a cooked vegetable.

Raspberries are a mind-boggling wellspring of numerous cancer prevention agents. They also contain manganese, supplement C, and dietary fiber. Verification recommends that the cell antioxidants present in raspberries may help pummel certain disease cells.

For example, in one lab study, analysts found that the cell antioxidants and some unique blends in raspberries helped slaughter chest, colon, and stomach infection cells in a test tube.

By virtue of chest malady, the pros credited some 50% of the malignant growth cell annihilation to the antioxidants effects of the raspberry remove.

A later audit of studies demonstrated that the mixes in black raspberries might slow the movement of harmful tumors.

Notwithstanding, the vast majority of the study on raspberries has included analyses in test tubes. Subsequently, specialists need to complete a study, including individuals to pass judgment on the viability of eating raspberries in forestalling illness.

8. Beans

Research has exhibited that pinto beans could help in smothering sorts of cancer.

Beans are an amazing source of protein and dietary fiber. A couple of beans, for instance, pinto beans, are also high in antioxidants.

Pinto beans contain a plant flavonoid called kaempferol, which may help smother cancer improvement and diminish the irritation. A couple of study interface kaempferol to the covering of unequivocal malignancies, including:

- bosom
- lung
- bladder
- kidney

In spite of these promising investigations, analysts don't contemplate the antioxidant effect of kaempferol in individuals. Until this point, they have essentially done a study in creatures and test tubes.

Nonetheless, as beans have a few potential medical advantages, it is a smart thought for individuals to incorporate them as a major aspect of their standard eating diet.

9. Purple or red grapes

Purple and red grape varieties contain supplement C, selenium, and antioxidants.

Two of the antioxidants agents that occur in grapes, explicitly proanthocyanin, and anthocyanin may help shield a person from heart sickness or infection.

Regardless, there is a necessity for additional examination to show the particular effects that eating grapes has on heart wellbeing and cancer hazard.

10. Spinach

Spinach is a green, verdant vegetable overflowing with supplements, minerals, and antioxidants. It is low in calories, choosing it an incredible choice as a development to servings of salad.

Lutein and zeaxanthin are two of the antioxidants in spinach that may propel eye wellbeing. They assist keep with hurting from brilliant (UV) pillars and other ruinous light waves.

A review of studies on zeaxanthin and lutein saw that lots of studies had investigated their activity in age-related macular degeneration. The authors, in the like manner, suggested how people could get a more prominent measure of these antioxidants in their weight control plans, naming dark verdant greens, eggs, and pistachios as sources.

11. Beets

Beets are vegetables that contain antioxidants having a spot with a class of shades called betalains. Betalains may help hinder cancer and stomach related issues.

Beets are similarly a wellspring of dietary fiber, folate, iron, and potassium. These substances may help with smothering disturbance.

One review saw that betalains show an assurance for decreasing free radicals and thwarting infection. Nevertheless, ask about has not yet chosen the practicality of eating beets for these focal points.

12. Kale

Kale is rich in supplements A, C, and K, and it contains a couple of antioxidants. It is a notable health food and extreme winter vegetable, typical in numerous northern zones.

Red kale offers more than green kale since it contains anthocyanins.

Anthocyanin are antioxidants that are quickly available in a variety of nourishments developed starting from the earliest stage. They are liable for the shade of these nourishments, from enthusiastic red to blue.

13. Orange vegetables

A couple of orange vegetables contain supplements and various supplements. These vegetables contain a lot of phytochemicals that can help with heart disease and malignancy neutralization. A couple of examples of orange vegetables with high cell reinforcement levels include:

- acorn squash
- butternut squash
- sweet potatoes
- carrots

There are obliged confirmation to prescribe how best to serve orange vegetables. Normally, people cook them; however, an individual can eat a couple of varieties, for instance, carrots or salad.

Summary

There are quite many customary types of nourishment that people can eat to build the number of cell antioxidants that they use.

The antioxidants in these nourishments may help advance eye health and heart, cancer, and guarantee against other fundamental infections that researchers with destructive free radicals.

In any case, researchers, despite everything, need to comprehend the degree to which every one of these nourishments assists individuals with procuring more elevated levels of antioxidants. They likewise need to decide how successful each is in infection anticipation.

CHAPTER FOUR
QUICK AND TASTY IMMUNITY RECIPES

1. GO TO THE MEDITERRANEAN

By keeping your body well-fed with a healthy and balanced diet; you can literally "eat well."

Nutrients are needed for every part of the immune system and renewal, repair, and defense from infections and disease. So, your strength will depend on the quality of your diet. Therefore, it is vital to maintain a healthy and balanced diet that provides an adequate supply of vitamins, minerals, and dietary fiber.

But what is a healthy and balanced diet? Studies have shown that the so-called "Mediterranean diet" can offer protection against obesity, heart disease, osteoporosis, cancer, and diabetes.

The Mediterranean diet is rich in fruit, vegetables, and whole grains. It contains adequate quantities of bluefish, nuts, seeds, legumes, dairy products, lean meat, or meat substitutes. The consumption rate of saturated fat, salt, and sugar should be reduced, and refined and processed foods are completely off the menu. Olive oil, the primary source of fat in the Mediterranean diet, is an excellent source of monounsaturated fatty acids that help reduce cholesterol. It is also rich in vitamins and antioxidants that fight cancer and reduce the risk of developing degenerative diseases.

In a nutshell, research suggests that the Mediterranean diet, with its emphasis on a wide variety of fresh whole foods, and the odd glass of antioxidant-rich red wine, is the model for a healthy diet that strengthens the immune system.

2. DOUBLETAKE

The nutritional benefit you receive from fruits and vegetables is unmatched. It is highly recommended to eat five to nine servings of fruit and vegetables a day; one way to maximize the variety of vitamins, minerals, fiber, and antioxidants that boost the immune system is to make sure you eat two different colors of fruit and vegetables with every meal.

Each different-colored fruit and vegetable contains unique healthy components that are essential for our health. The phrase "eat a rainbow of fruit and vegetables" is an easy way to remember getting as many colors as possible so that you can maximize your intake of a wide range of nutrients.

Red: tomatoes, berries, peppers, and radishes contain nutrients that can reduce the risk of prostate cancer, lower blood pressure, reduce tumor growth and cholesterol levels, eliminate harmful free radicals and support joint tissue in case of arthritis.

Orange and yellow: carrots, sweet potatoes, pumpkin, oranges, papaya, and other orange and yellow fruits and vegetables contain nutrients that can reduce age-related macular degeneration and the risk of prostate cancer, reduce cholesterol and blood pressure, promote the formation of collagen and healthy joints. It fights harmful free radicals and works with magnesium and calcium to build healthy bones.

White: mushrooms, pakchoi, and pumpkins contain nutrients that can activate the natural killer B and T cells, reduce the risk of colon, breast, and prostate cancers and balance hormone levels, reducing the risk of cancer-related to hormones.

Green: cabbage, spinach, cabbage, alfalfa sprouts, mustard, and cabbage are examples of green vegetables that contain nutrients that can reduce the risk of cancer, lower blood pressure, and lower cholesterol levels. Increase digestion, support retinal health and vision, combat harmful radical damage, and increase the immune system's activity.

Blue and purple: cranberries, pomegranates, grapes, elderberries, aubergines, and plums contain nutrients that stimulate healthy digestion and act as carcinogens in the digestive tract.

3. DRINK YOUR LEMONS

Drinking a glass of lemon juice diluted with filtered water every morning is the perfect way to start digestion and increase immunity at the same time. Lemons fruits contain bioflavonoids, a group of nutrients that increase immunity by protecting the body's cells from environmental pollutants.

The receptor sites found in the microscopic parking spaces along the membrane of each cell housed Contaminants. Such as toxins or germs that can park here and gradually reach the cell membrane. Still, when bioflavonoids fill these parking lots, there is no room to park toxins. Bioflavonoids also reduce the cholesterol's ability to form plaques in the arteries and decrease the formation of microscopic arterial blood clots, which can cause heart attacks and strokes. Research has proven that people who consume more bioflavonoids have minimal cardiovascular disease.

Lemon is also the ideal food to restore the acid-alkaline balance in your body. Drinking freshly squeezed lemon juice in water first in the morning or adding it to tea, salad dressings (instead of vinegar), cooking or cooking, helps maintain your body's internal balance at a pH that supports healthy bacteria instead of harmful viruses and bacteria that thrive in more acidic environments. Apple cider vinegar is another excellent way to improve your body's alkalinity. Still, the taste of lemons is much more delightful!

Drinking fresh lemon juice To prepare a glass of fresh lemon juice, squeeze the juice of one lemon into a glass, add 300 ml of slightly warm filtered water, and one teaspoon of maple syrup for sweetness. Mix and drink immediately. Remember, the first thing in the morning, about fifteen minutes before breakfast, is the optimal time to drink lemon juice.

4. ALKALI, ALKALI, ALKALI

Your immune system is stronger in an alkaline environment. Many bacteria and viruses love an acidic environment, but cannot survive in a healthy alkaline state. If you feel exhausted, eating lots of green vegetables and drinking lots of water will increase alkalinity and, therefore, your immunity.

Your immune system is dependent on water. It transports nutrients to cells, transports wastes, bacteria, toxins out of cells and out of the body, maintains body temperature stability, protects joints, and keeps the lining of the mouth hydrated and moist, reducing susceptibility to colds. Don't wait until you're thirsty to drink water, as well as thirst, along with headaches and dark yellow urine (healthy urine is pale yellow), a sign of dehydration. Your body's need for water is constant, and experts recommend drinking six to eight glasses a day, more if you're sweating, exercising, or getting hot. And it is better to drink only filtered water since tap water can be contaminated with lead and other toxins that your body doesn't want or need.

5. ONE YOGURT PER DAY

Look for yogurt that contains active crops that indicate useful bacteria and try eating one every day for breakfast or dessert, or use live yogurt in salad dressings, smoothies and sauces. Live white yogurt a day can help keep infections at bay. This is because these yogurts contain probiotics, bacteria that stimulate immune cells in the gastrointestinal (GI) tract.

The regular and healthy bacteria that colonize the gastrointestinal tract help you resist bad bacteria and detoxify harmful substances. In addition to its protective effect on the gastrointestinal tract, probiotics can also help stimulate the production of immune cells throughout the system. In recent research, the University of Vienna, those who ate yogurt every day for two weeks, increased the T lymphocyte cell count, which enhances the immune system by nearly 30 percent.

6. FOS POWER

A bowl of porridge or chopped wheat for breakfast will provide your immune system with a much needed prebiotic solution. We need pre and probiotics in our bodies. Probiotics are many and varied. The most commonly known is called Lactobacillus acidophilus, which is found in bright white yogurt, but more and more are discovered.

Prebiotics, also known as FOS (fruit-oligo-saccharides) is a type of natural fiber that nourishes and supports the excellent work of friendly or probiotic bacteria. Prebiotics are natural elements found in foods such as garlic, onion, leek, shallot, asparagus, spinach, Jerusalem artichoke, chicory, peas, beans, lentils, oats, and bananas. Therefore, including more of these foods in the diet will increase both the digestive system and immunity. One of the best ways to make sure you have enough FOS power in your diet to eat oatmeal, grated wheat, or other whole breakfast cereals.

7. GOOD COFFEE HABITS

Coffee doesn't help the immune system to do its job efficiently, so cut your coffee intake down to no more than two cups a day.

Caffeine in coffee can temporarily increase alertness, improve performance, and perhaps even improve concentration. But, experts say it's important to remember that the main ingredient in coffee, caffeine is a drug before pouring you another cup. It is not a nutrient necessary for good health, such as vitamins and minerals. Caffeine can also dehydrate you and remove essential nutrients that stimulate the immune system from your body, such as calcium, which stimulates the bones. Too much caffeine can also cause health problems, such as hypertension, brittle bones, sleep disturbances, and irritability.

You don't have to quit drinking coffee, but if you drink more than three cups of coffee a day, you should reduce it to one or two cups. Here are some tips to make sure your coffee drinking habits are healthy:
- When you drink your coffee, be sure to add a glass of water to your daily water intake per cup of coffee to avoid its dehydrating effects.

- On average, Drink one to three cups of coffee per day (up to 300 mg of caffeine) does not seem to have any adverse effect on most healthy people. However, pregnant women, children, people with heart disease or peptic ulcers, and the elderly may be more sensitive to caffeine's effects. Therefore it is recommended to limit their consumption.

- Keep in mind that the caffeine content in coffee varies widely depending on roasting and fermentation methods and the size of the cup used in drinking. For example, a recent study showed that a cup of 475 ml (16 floz) of house blend in a leading coffee chain had a massive average of 259 mg of caffeine.

- Replace some of the lost nutrients by adding two tablespoons of milk to your coffee or turning your espresso into milk.

Coffee is the primary source of caffeine for many people. Still, other items, such as soda, tea, chocolate, and cold and headache medications, also contain caffeine and can significantly increase the daily caffeine intake. As for chocolate (another source of caffeine), make sure that the type you eat is quality dark chocolate, containing at least 70% cocoa solids. Some people hear the hum of caffeine more than others.

Pay attention to your body system and know when to say "no" to that extra cup of coffee, even if you're surrounded by people who drink it like water. It is important to note that coffee drinkers who skip their daily dose may experience a temporary suspension of caffeine (usually in the form of a headache or drowsiness). Still, these symptoms will subside within 24-48 hours.

8. SUGAR OFF

The next time you are tempted to take a chocolate bar, drink a sweetened drink, or eat a sweetened cereal, pause your immune system and take a fruit or bowl of oatmeal.

The impact of refined white sugar on the immune system can be enormous. Eating or drinking eight tablespoons (100 grams) of sugar is the same quantity as two cans of a soda full of sugar, which can reduce the ability of white blood cells to kill germs by 40 percent. The immunosuppressive effect of sugar begins less than 30 minutes after ingestion and can last up to 5 hours. In addition to all this, a sugar-rich diet increases the risk of blood sugar imbalances, which can lead to mood swings, weight gain, fatigue, headache, hormonal imbalances, and a host of other unpleasant symptoms.

If you only do one thing to strengthen your immune system, removing the sugar will do the trick. Minimizing sugar consumption does some magic. Sugar doesn't give nutrients, only calories. So, a reduction in sugar consumption rate yields excellent results in your immunity, energy levels, and weight distribution, and the ability to think clearly when you break your appetite and stop eating refined sugar.

Reducing sugar intake may seem daunting initially, but it's easier than you think if you follow these tips for total sugar shutdown:

Sweet Substitutes: Try sugar-free fruit and fruit juices more often with meals and snacks to reduce sugar. Fruits have natural sugars, but they also give you essential vitamins and minerals. Plan to have fresh seasonal fruit for dessert. Use dried fruit to sweeten cereals and baked goods. Cut a banana or fresh peach instead of using jam on a peanut butter sandwich. Prepare your drinks with unsweetened fruit juice and sparkling water.

Pass the sugar: remove the sugar bowl from the table and, if you add sugar to the tea, gradually reduce it until you need it. Stick to this because once the taste buds get used to tea and other hot drinks without sugar, you will never want to go back. And by reducing, you also reduce the amount of sugar you use for baking.

Do not wholly ban sugar: a little sugar, added judiciously to healthy foods, can make them more appetizing, a pinch of brown sugar in oatmeal or grapefruit, or a teaspoon of maple syrup in the winter squash enhances the flavor of these healthy options. It is best to avoid sugar substitutes, as some studies suggest that they may also have adverse health effects.

Cereal Killer: Some breakfast cereals have four or more teaspoons of sugar added to each serving! When you buy sugar-free cereals, you can save money and add sweetener at home if you wish. Sprinkle the fresh, canned, or dried fruit over the cereals to sweeten them.

Read the labels: when you buy food, read the ingredient labels to find the quantity and types of sugars that have been added to the food. Many types of sugar are used to make sweet and crunchy food. Search for words ending with "dare" or "ol," such as dextrose, fructose, maltose, sucrose, glucose, lactose, mannitol, and sorbitol.

These are all forms of sugar. Syrups as sweeteners for corn, sorghum syrup, and high fructose syrups are sweeteners that are often added to drinks. Brown sugar, molasses, and honey can be "natural," but they give you all the same calories as refined table sugar. The ingredients are listed in order of weight. From highest to lowest, when a type of sugar or syrup is the first ingredient, you will know that there is more sugar than any other ingredient. Some foods can contain many types of sugar. If added together, the total can be more than any other ingredient in that food.

Switch from white bread, pasta and rice to whole grains - Whole grains are rich in nutrients and fiber that can keep your blood sugar and appetite levels balanced for hours after eating, unlike sugar, which gives you a high followed by a deep low.

9. CONQUER YOUR SWEET TOOTH

If you have a sweet tooth and always crave something sweet, you have to conquer it. A sugar-rich diet depresses the immune system and stops working efficiently. To overcome the sweet tooth, make sure to always have breakfast and never leave more than two or three hours between meals and snacks.

This is because eating little and often and speeding up the metabolism first is keeping your blood sugar levels balanced, making you less likely to want. Aim for a healthy breakfast,

71

followed by a satisfying mid-morning snack (a fruit and a handful of nuts and seeds, for example), a healthy lunch, a mid-afternoon snack, a dinner, and a light snack before going to bed.

For your blood sugar balance and appetite control, your meals and snacks should be a mixture of fiber-rich carbohydrates (such as whole grains, fruits, and vegetables) and healthy proteins (such as nuts, seeds, or products). Dairy) that they give you They offer your body and brain a prolonged release of energy to make you feel full.

Avoid sweets, cakes, chips, and other processed or refined foods; These give you a quick burst of energy followed by an extended, drawn bass. And finally, if the cravings hit you, try these sweet and energetic delicacies. They will be able to satisfy your treats and improve your health and immunity at the same time:

A spoon or two dried fruit: low in fat and low glycemic index, which means that they slowly absorb from the stomach into the bloodstream and make you feel full longer. Dried fruits are also rich in iron and fiber, increasing immunity and energy.

Berry mix: The mixture of blueberries, raspberries, blackberries, and cherries in a large bowl is a very healthy fruit snack. It is low in fat and contains many vitamins and bioflavonoids, which can increase immunity. You could also add some low-fat, calcium-rich yogurt that develops bones.

Fruit milkshake:

A low-fat, energizing, and nutrient-rich snack that tastes delicious.

10. RED, RED WINE

Enjoy a small glass of red wine with your meal. Recent studies show that drinking no more than one glass of red wine a day can have some immune strengthening benefits by protecting against certain types of cancer and heart disease and can have a positive effect on cholesterol levels and blood pressure.

Drinking wine with food and being suitable for the heart, can also help prevent food poisoning before it occurs. Oregon State University scientists recently discovered that wine could bring out three common food pathogens: E. coli, listeria, and salmonella. In laboratory studies, the combination of ethanol and organic acids in wine seemed to mix the genetic material of insects.

All wines have a similar effect, say the researchers, but reds are the most powerful. Drinking excess of excess, however, does not produce the same benefits. Excessive alcohol consumption can damage the immune system in two ways. First, it creates a general nutritional deficiency, depriving the body of valuable nutrients that stimulate the immune system.

Secondly, alcohol, like sugar, consumed in excess can reduce the ability of white blood cells to kill germs. High doses of alcohol suppress the ability of white blood cells to multiply. It inhibits the action of killer white blood cells on cancer cells. It decreases the ability of immune cells called macrophages to produce the tumor necrosis factor that kills cancer cells.

A drink (the equivalent of 350 ml (12 floz) of beer, 150 ml (5 floz) of wine or 25 ml (1 floz) of alcohol does not appear to disturb the immune system, but three or more drinks do damage to the immune system increases in proportion to the amount of alcohol consumed, so if you are tempted to buy another round, remember that the quantities of alcohol that are sufficient to cause poisoning are also sufficient to suppress immunity.

11. RAW POWER

Reduce the amount of cooking you cook, because cooked foods, especially overcooked ones, decrease the number of nutrients that strengthen the immune system. This doesn't mean you shouldn't cook at all. Some foods, such as eggs, meat, and fish, can be dangerous when raw and must be well prepared. Try balancing cooked food with raw food, perhaps 50:50, and cook gently, at a lower temperature and longer if necessary.

(It is always better to avoid aluminum pans, as this can increase the toxic load on the immune system.) Steaming is the ideal way to cook vegetables, frying is an excellent way to cook fish, and poaching is useful for eggs and fish. Meat should be roasted as other methods, such as frying, use too much fat.

So, without going overboard. Eat something raw with each meal or start each meal with something natural, such as an apple for breakfast and a stalk of celery or chopped cucumber for lunch or dinner.

12. FEEL THE BURN

A curry once or twice a week can refresh the taste buds and the immune system. Enjoying a curry every week or a pinch or two of spicy sauce with meals could help keep insects at bay. Various animal and laboratory studies have shown that capsaicin, the compound that sets chili peppers on fire, can help stop the disease before it starts.

In one study, the mice received a daily dose of capsaicin. After three weeks, they had three times more antibody-producing cells than those without capsaicin. More antibodies mean fewer colds and infections. The results of other studies suggest that eating foods containing hot components such as capsaicin can improve immunity by eliminating toxins.

So, if you like spicy and hot foods, go ahead and treat yourself. Curry is fast approaching fish and chips as the UK's most popular takeaway. To make a healthy choice for your home cooking, ensure the fresh use of curry as the fresh curry are rich and free of additives.

13. PROTEINS FULL OF ENERGY

Taste some lean protein with every meal. The amino acids found in proteins form the building blocks of all cells in the body, including the cells that feed the immune system. Shortage in the consumption of food with a lower protein leads to fewer white blood cells to fight disease-causing antigens.

One of the ways that immune cells fight pathogens is by increasing their numbers. Proteins and amino acids are vital to stimulate the proliferation of immune cells. Besides, proteins help maintain blood sugar balance and an alkaline immune status. Low protein diets also tend to be rich in carbohydrates, especially refined carbohydrates, which easily convert to glucose, increase blood sugar, and put a strain on the pancreas and immune system.

Your body cannot store proteins. As it contains carbohydrates and fats, it needs a constant supply; consequently, you should try eating good quality protein with every meal and snack. But remember that quality matters. To avoid the health risks of saturated fat, choose 3 to 4 ounces (75 to 125 g) portions of lean proteins, such as fish, shellfish, poultry (without skin), eggs, lentils, and legumes and soy products. Other significant sources of protein include dairy products, wheat germ, and spirulina, cereals such as quinoa, green leafy vegetables, peas, nuts, seeds, see-weed, and Quorn.

Don't overdo it, as a protein-rich diet can increase the risk of diabetes and heart disease. Also, it is important to eat little with meal and snack., you must also eat nutritious and healthy carbohydrates and fats as part of a varied and balanced diet. Try to get around 25 percent of your total daily calorie intake from protein sources; 20-25 percent of healthy fats and the rest of carbohydrates in the form of whole grains, fruits, and vegetables.

14. GET OUT OF YOUR WHEY

Sprinkle some whey protein powder that boosts the immune system in your smoothies or yogurt. An impressive range of benefits can be derived from consuming whey protein. Most of us don't know about it. When it increases weight loss and cardiovascular health, whey protein can also support the immune system and increase bone mineral density.

Adding whey protein to your diet is a powerful way to increase your immunity. This is because whey proteins are rich in an amino acid called cysteine, which is converted into glutathione in the body. Glutathione is a powerful antioxidant that strengthens cells against bacterial or viral infections. For maximum protein concentration, try whey protein isolate powder, which is purer and slightly more expensive than concentrate?

Strengthen your morning smoothie with whey protein powder or try another source: bright white yogurt. The clear liquid that forms over most yogurt cartons is pure whey protein, so don't drain it, but add it to the yogurt.

Fruit Whey Protein Shake
- 125 g (4 ounces) of pure white yogurt
- 125–200 ml (4–7 floz) of water

- 100 g (3 ^{1} / 2 oz) of fresh or frozen berries
- One (1) medium banana
- One (1) tablespoon of whey protein powder
- 2 or 3 ice cubes (not necessary if using frozen fruit)

Put all the ingredients in a blender and whisk until smooth.

White Yogurt with Whey Powder

- One (1) tablespoon of whey protein powder
- 125 g (4 ounces) of pure white yogurt
- ^{1} / 2 teaspoons of honey

Sprinkle with cinnamon to decorate

Stir the whey protein powder into a bowl of bright white yogurt. Add the honey and add the cinnamon chips.

15. ANTIOXIDANT PROTECTIONS ON A PLATE

Store antioxidant-rich foods and your immune system will be strengthened day after day.

Antioxidants are a group of vitamins, minerals, and unique compounds with incredible immunostimulant benefits, which protect cells from free radical damage. Free radicals in your body system can cause cell damage. The damage can lead to diseases. They are produced by all types of combustion: environmental pollution, smoke, radiation, fried foods (high levels of heat damage the oil). Fortunately, nature provides us with rich sources of antioxidant nutrients to break down free radicals and offers instant protection on a plate.

Vitamin A, beta carotene, vitamin C, vitamin E, zinc, and selenium antioxidants are essential in our diet. These antioxidants help to protect our system from free radical damage. Among all these antioxidants, vitamin C is king, as it is antibacterial and antiviral, and it is a natural antihistamine that helps in the body's response to allergens. Each day, eating six servings of fresh fruit and vegetables will give you about 200 mg of vitamin C (the recommended daily allowance). High-level sources of vitamin C include citrus fruits, kiwis, papayas, strawberries, black currants, green vegetables, tomatoes, potatoes, broccoli, red and green peppers parsley.

To make sure you have enough antioxidant protection, try making the snack fruitful, add more fruits and vegetables to your kitchen, and get into the habit of serving two vegetables with your meals instead of one. And don't forget that smoothies and fruit and vegetable juices also count.

16. ONE CARROT PER DAY

Many of us grow up listening to "eat your carrots; they will help you see in the dark." You might think it's just one of those old wives' stories, but scientific research has shown that the story is true. It's not just your night vision that carrots can improve. Eating a rich carrot Beta carotene before or after a meal can do more than refresh your breath and brighten your eyesight. In essence, it can feed your immune system.

Studies have shown that beta carotene antioxidants can reduce the risk of cardiovascular disease, particularly stroke and heart attack, by providing scientific support for the belief that one carrot per day can keep the heart surgeon away. Beta-carotene also protects against cancer by stimulating immune cells called macrophages to produce the tumor necrosis factor, which kills cancer cells.

Fruits and vegetables are found to contain Beta-carotene. It is available in yellow and orange fruits and vegetables such as carrots, tomatoes, mangoes, sweet potatoes, red and yellow peppers, and dark green vegetables such as spinach, watercress, and broccoli.

Carrot Soup That Increases Immunity

- One (1) tablespoon of extra virgin olive oil
- One (1) medium onion, chopped
- Seven (7) large carrots, washed, peeled and chopped
- One (1) inch (2.5 cm) fresh ginger root, chopped
- One (1) cube of vegetable broth
- 900 ml (1 1 / 2 pints) of boiling water
- One (1) teaspoon freshly ground black pepper
- One (1) tablespoon of fresh basil to decorate sea salt, to taste

1. Heat the oil in a large pan. Add onion, carrots, and ginger and cook for five minutes to soften.

2. In a separate measuring spoon, prepare the vegetable broth using boiling water and the cube of broth. Add to the pan and bring to a boil. Cover the saucepan and simmer for 35 minutes or until the carrots are tender.

3. Pour the measured quantity in the pan into a food processor or blender. Add black pepper and blitz to obtain a homogeneous consistency, adding more water if necessary. It may be required to do it in two lots.

4. Return the soup to the pan and heat gently. Check the seasoning, then garnish with basil and serve.

17. DRESS FOR SUCCESS

while you prepare your salad at home, add a generous portion of olive oil or walnuts to the dressing. Eating salad is a smart food choice for lunch or dinner, but don't dip it with fat-free condiments.

A study conducted at Iowa State University found that without fat in the diet, your body does not absorb some of the nutrients that fight disease in vegetables. The researchers fed seven people with salad for twelve weeks and tested the blood after each meal. Those who supplemented their salads with fat-free dressings failed to consistently absorb carotenoids (antioxidants that have been linked to better immunity).

Fat is necessary for carotenoids to reach absorbent intestinal cells, so be sure to choose medications based on healthy fats such as extra virgin olive oil, sunflower oil, or flaxseed oil. And if you're feeling adventurous, try dressing. Don't just stick with the proven olive oil. Experiment with other types of healthy oil such as sunflower, sesame, and nut oil.

18 PUT SEZ ON YOUR PLATE

Vitamin C and vitamin A are not the only antioxidants that increase your immunity. To get your full portion of antioxidant protection, you need to make sure you put enough SEZ (selenium, vitamin E, and zinc) on your plate every day.

- Selenium increases natural killer cells and mobilizes cancer cells. Good food sources include nuts (especially Brazil nuts), seeds, whole grains, shellfish, egg yolks, sunflower seeds, and garlic.
- Vitamin E increases the production of natural killer cells that hunt and destroy unwanted viruses, bacteria, and cancer cells. Good food sources of vitamin E are avocados, nuts, seeds, unrefined oils, and oats.
- Having sufficient zinc in our body help to speed up the growth of white blood cells that stimulate the immune system, especially lymphocytes. Good food sources include lean meat, ginger, pumpkin seeds, Brazil nuts, and whole grains.

19.IRON ORE

Eating some iron-rich nuts, such as raisins, during the day will strengthen the immune system. Iron is a mineral necessary for the production of white blood cells and antibodies, and without sufficient iron, it is more likely that colds and frequent infections will occur.

A low iron diet can also increase the risk of anemia, a condition in which red blood cells do not supply adequate oxygen to the body's tissues. Symptoms include fatigue, shortness of breath, and bleeding gums. The best sources of dietary iron are lean red meat, seafood (such as lake trout, clams, and oysters), eggs, legumes (such as beans, peas, and lentils), nuts, seeds, whole grains, dried fruit, and leafy vegetables green and iron-enriched cereals and pasta.

Non-meat iron sources are more natural to absorb when combined with a good source of vitamin C, such as citrus or fruit juice, berries, peppers, broccoli, cabbage, tomatoes, Brussels sprouts, melon, kiwi, mango and papaya.

Iron-Rich Vegetable Juice Recipe

- One (1) glass of filtered water
- One (1) beetroot, washed and finely chopped
- Two (2) carrots, washed, peeled and finely chopped
- Two (2) tomatoes, washed, peeled and finely chopped
- Three (3) fresh spinach leaves, washed and finely chopped
- Juice of lime or fresh lemon to facilitate absorption (first add a few drops, then add others to taste)
- A pinch of black pepper

1. To prepare this healthy morning drink, put all the ingredients in a blender.

2. Cover and treat until smooth. Serve immediately

20. OTHER OMEGA-3

Eating bluefish at least once a week, but no more than three times a week is an effective way to strengthen the immune system. A high-fat diet can damage the immune system by decreasing the function of T lymphocytes. Saturated fat (found in animal products and fried foods) can contribute to heart disease and weight gain. In contrast, Trans fats (found in margarine and many commercial baked goods) can contribute to low-grade chronic inflammation in the body. Therefore, limit your fat intake to 30 percent of your daily calorie intake, with saturated fats from 5 to 10 percent.

For the remaining 20-25 percent, look for sources of unsaturated fats, such as canola oil, olive oil, walnuts, avocados, and seeds. Increase your consumption of omega-3 fatty acids in your body system—this helps to fight inflammation and free the immune system to defend itself against antigens. Well documented for their ability to protect us from heart disease, omega-3 fatty acids are found in oily fish such as mackerel, sardines, salmon, trout, and fresh tuna (but not canned tuna). They help immunity by stimulating the activity of white blood cells that attack bacteria.

A recent study found that children who took half a teaspoon of linseed oil each day had fewer and less severe respiratory infections and fewer days of absence from school. The omega-3 fatty acids contained in linseed oil and fatty fish act as immune stimulators by increasing the activity of phagocytes, the white blood cells that bacteria eat. (Maybe that's why grandmothers insisted on a daily dose of lousy cod liver oil.) Essential fatty acids also protect the body from damage caused by excessive reactions to infections.

If you are a vegetarian or don't like fish, you can increase the intake of this micronutrient by incorporating linseed oil into your diet. An easy way to get more omega-3 fatty acids into your diet is to add 1-3 teaspoons of linseed oil to a smoothie and yogurt, or salads, or other dishes. Oil loses nutrients when heated, so it's best to eat it cold.

21. MAINTAIN AN ENERGY BALANCE

Your immune system works best when you consume enough food calories, not too many or too few per day. Excessive calorie consumption can have harmful effects on cellular production in the immune system by increasing the production of compounds called prostaglandins, which have a suppressive effect on the production of T lymphocytes. Fewer T cells patrolling the body increase the odds. For an antigen to catch on.

On the other hand, low-calorie consumption can be just as damaging. Considerable evidence shows that diets, anorexia, or nutritional deficiencies increase a person's susceptibility to infections. Following a low-calorie diet or spending long periods without eating is a surefire way to reduce immunity. This is because if you starve, your body will think it is under siege and will pump stress hormones that disturb blood sugar levels and harm immunity.

Besides, losing more than 1 kg (2.2 lbs) per week is difficult for T cells to detect diseased or foreign cells. Studies have shown that the best and most effective way to lose weight if you have weight is to lose it gradually. A 2007 study at the University of California to date, the world's largest research on weight loss, has shown that dieting is harmful because of the tendency of the diet to lose and therefore regain the weight. ; This yo-yo diet effect increases the risk of heart attacks, strokes, and diabetes. Starving or depriving the body of the nutrients needed to boost immunity and metabolism (fat burning), therefore, will not only increase your chances of succumbing to colds or flu but will inevitably also lead to an increase in your weight back directly.

Being overweight can weaken immunity, but don't try to remedy by following a strict diet, as this could make things worse. If you have weight to lose, look for a loss of no more than $1/2$–1 kg (1 2 lb) per week and maintain vital energy balance by eating healthy and increasing the amount of exercise you do.

22. EGGS ARE EASY

Eating an egg for breakfast every day is a great way to increase energy levels and be sure to take a dose of magnesium that strengthens the immune system. Calcium is known for its importance for building strong and healthy bones, but less about the importance of eating enough magnesium-rich foods, your partner that stimulates the immune system.

Magnesium is needed for antibody protection, and low magnesium levels can increase the risk of allergic reactions because a deficiency of magnesium can increase histamine levels. Good food sources include nuts, seeds, green leafy vegetables, tubers, egg yolks, whole grains, and dried fruit. Calcium and magnesium are not only crucial for increasing immunity, but they cannot function well without one another. This is because magnesium helps your body absorb calcium, so even if your diet is high in calcium, it can be deficient if you are not eating enough magnesium-rich foods.

23. PUT THE KETTLE ON

Your immune system receives a natural boost whenever you lift your feet and enjoy a cup of tea. Many studies support the view that tea is good for health. Scientists tend to agree that tea, both black and green, can make a positive contribution to promoting health and preventing chronic diseases.

Recent research has revealed that the antioxidants in tea can inhibit the growth of cancer cells, support dental health, increase bone density, and strengthen cardiovascular health. According to a recent study, heart attack patients who drank tea reduced their risk of death by up to 44 percent compared to those who did not drink tea. There is no evidence that tea has dehydrated or that consumption of three or four cups a day. It was harmful to health. They recommended it positively. Research, however, suggests that tea can affect the body's ability to absorb iron from food, indicating that people at risk of anemia should avoid drinking tea with meals.

24. THE MAGIC OF GARLIC

Add a touch of immunostimulating magic to your diet by cooking or preparing your meal with garlic. A member of the allium family known for centuries is the garlic. It is very popular among different cultures for its protective properties. This tasty ingredient acts as a powerful immune enhancer that stimulates the multiplication of white blood cells that fight infections, increases the natural activity of killer cells, and increases the efficiency of antibody production.

The immunostimulating properties of garlic seem to be due to its sulfur-containing compounds, such as allicin and sulphides, which give garlic its characteristic flavor. Garlic also acts as an antioxidant which reduces the accumulation of free radicals in the bloodstream and plays a role in the elimination of possible carcinogens and other toxic substances; Proof of this is that crops with a garlic-rich diet have a lower incidence of bowel cancer. It is also a food for the heart, as it prevents platelets from sticking and blocking small blood vessels.

Mash the garlic in the stews, roast them together with the meat or mash them with avocado and lemon juice to make an immune stew. If you don't like the taste of garlic (or are concerned about the breath that smells like garlic), try the odorless and tasteless capsule form now available in health food stores.

Garlic Bread

- One (1) loaf of French bread
- (125 g) 4 ounces of unsalted butter
- (50 g) 2 oz fresh parsley, finely chopped

- Two (2) large garlic cloves, finely chopped paprika (optional)

1. Cut the bread into 1-inch thick slices, but not completely.
2. Combine butter, parsley, and garlic, mixing well.
3. Distribute between the slices of bread and sprinkle with paprika, if desired.
4. Reassemble the bread, wrap it in aluminum foil and bake for 20 minutes at 180 ° C (350 ° F).

25. GREEN LEAF DEFENSE

Green leafy vegetables rich in antioxidant power include cabbage, broccoli, and spinach. It strengthens the immune system and fights cancer. Make sure to eat your vegetables every day or every other day. Spinach is rich in carotenoids, which the body converts to vitamin A to promote the immune response.

The vitamin C content of spinach keeps the skin and mucous membranes healthy, while its vitamin B content increases energy. Spinach is also an excellent source of zinc, needed to promote T cell activity. Try this hot pot that stimulates the immune system.

Spinach And Baked Potatoes

- 300 g of spinach
- 150 g of fresh cream
- Two (2) tablespoons of granulated mustard
- One (1) clove of garlic, crushed
- 750 (1 $\frac{1}{2}$ lb) of potatoes, peeled and cut into thin slices

1. Steam the spinach, drain well and finely chop.
2. Mix the fresh cream with the mustard and the crushed garlic clove.
3. Use a third of the potato to cover the base of a baking sheet, then put half of the spinach on top of the potato and pour some of the cream mixtures.
4. Add another layer of previous content with a layer of potato and fresh cream mixture as the last ingredient.

5. Cover with aluminum foil and cook for one hour at 180 ° C (350 ° F) Gas 4.

6. Remove the foil and cook for another 20 minutes or until tender and lightly browned.

26. BRIGHT BERRIES

All berries are bright to increase immunity because they are rich in vitamin C, but in particular black currants and blueberries stand out. Black currant contains nutrients that can improve iron absorption, increase metabolism, and improve oxygen transport to tissues. They help liver function, help regulate blood sugar levels, and stimulate wound healing. They can also offer protection against heart disease and cancer.

Blueberries are among the richest sources of anti-aging antioxidants that stimulate the immune system and cancer and scientists have found that they have many other health benefits, such as improving brain function and balancing sugar levels in the body. Blood. Try this berry-based immune smoothie, which also contains apples (apples contain pectin, which has anti-cancer properties; they are also rich in vitamin C, calcium, magnesium and beta-carotene and can help flush out the liver and kidneys):

Bright Berry Smoothie

- One (1) large apple
- 150 ml of pure white yogurt
- Eight (8) berries
- Eight (8) blueberries
- Eight (8) raspberries
- A handful of organic oatmeal
- One (1) teaspoon maple syrup (optional)

1. Squeeze the apple juice and put it with the yogurt in a blender.

2. Add the berries and stir until smooth.

3. Pour into a shallow glass and sprinkle the oatmeal with an optional maple syrup thread over the oatmeal.

4. For a swirling effect, hold half of the yogurt and stir gently after mixing it until it is marbled.

27. AVOCADO FULL OF ENERGY

To strengthen your immune system, cut some avocado on your sandwiches and salads. Avocado is full of energy and phytochemicals that boost the immune system, helping protect against certain types of cancer. A rich source of antioxidants for the skin, it also helps stabilize blood sugar and blood pressure. It is a good source of vitamin C, vitamin E, and B6.

Avocado Salad

- Two (2) avocados
- Romaine lettuce leaves
- 1 / 2 teaspoons of black pepper
- 1 / 2 teaspoons of dried oregano
- One (1) clove of minced garlic
- One (1) sprig of fresh thyme
- 4–5 tablespoons of extra virgin olive oil
- One (1) tablespoon of red wine; 1 tablespoon of vinegar

1. Cut the avocados in half and discard the stone. Collect the avocado pulp with a scoop of ice cream and roll it into balls. Place them on two plates lined with lettuce leaves.

2. In a small bowl, mix the rest of the ingredients, pour over the avocados, and serve.

28. SEE RED

Tomatoes are rich in antioxidants, including vitamins A and C, along with lycopene, which can improve immune response, increase resistance to infectious diseases, promote wound healing, and keep skin and muscles in good condition. The American Journal of Clinical Nutrition, ten subjects followed a tomato-rich diet for three weeks, followed by a tomato-free diet for another three weeks.

While subjects were following the tomato diet, their white blood cells that fought infections suffered 38% less free radical damage (atoms in the body that damage and destabilize cells) than when they did not eat tomato products. Researchers speculate that lycopene in tomatoes acts as an antioxidant, helping white blood cells to resist the harmful effects of free radicals. Try baked tomatoes (or beans and tomatoes) on whole toast and homemade tomato soup. Don't forget that tomato ketchup, if used sparingly, is also a source of lycopene that strengthens the immune system.

29. INSTANT PROTECTION

Whenever you include the following foods in your food or kitchen, it immediately boosts your immune system.

Cinnamon: This culinary spice has wonderful antibacterial and antifungal properties. To prepare a hot toddy, fill a cup with boiling water and add two teaspoons of tea tree honey, a lemon juice, and a quarter of a cinnamon stick. Leave the drink to rest for 10 minutes, then remove the cinnamon stick; Relax and enjoy.

Nuts and seeds: A handful of nuts and seeds can be used as a snack between meals or sprinkled on your salad or soup. This will give your immune system a healthy dose of protein, zinc, B vitamins, vitamin E, selenium, magnesium, and essential fats. An example of nut reach in selenium is Brazil nuts. Almonds, hazelnuts, and sunflower seeds are best for vitamin E. In contrast, flax seeds are unique for omega-3s, sunflower seeds for omega-6s, proteins, and B vitamins and seeds squash are a particularly good source of zinc, necessary for healthy skin and the function of white blood cells.

Parsley: Parsley is a must for any refrigerator or window because it is rich in vitamins A and C, as well as magnesium and chlorophyll to fight cancer.

See-weed: A lot of minerals, vitamins, and amino acids are found in see-weed, so try adding some to your soups or mixing with mashed potatoes.

Shiitake Mushrooms - Excellent in stews, soups, and fried potatoes, Shiitake mushrooms have antibacterial, antiviral and anti-parasitic properties and are a natural source of protection against viruses.

SweetPotato: A rich source of vitamin E, sweet potato can contribute to heart health and is a good source of food antioxidants. It can help regulate high blood pressure, and its content of vitamin A and carotenoids can protect against inflammatory conditions. Why not try sweet potato puree or sweet potato curry?

30. BRIGHTER BREAKFAST SMOOTHIE

Give your immune system and your health the first shot of energy in the morning with this lively and energizing smoothie. This tropical fruit smoothie is just what helps strengthen the immune system. Few people are aware of the high levels of vitamin C found in kiwis. In fact, in terms of weight, kiwifruit contains twice as much vitamin C as oranges.

Kiwis smoothie is a good source of potassium, which can help maintain a healthy heart. Mangoes are a good source of vitamin C and carotenoids, both of which help strengthen the immune system. The softness of coconut milk helps balance the acidity of the kiwi. Spirulina is a blue-green see-weed of green sea-weed that contains nutrients that can strengthen the immune system. It has acquired importance as a green superfood of nature thanks to its rich concentration of perfectly balanced amino acids (proteins), fiber, vitamins, minerals, and other essential nutrients.

Smoothie for breakfast

- Two (2) kiwis, peeled and chopped
- One (1) mango or one nectarine, peeled, chopped and toned
- 100 ml (3 $\frac{1}{2}$ floz) of coconut milk
- Two (2) teaspoons of spirulina powder
- Three (3) fluid ounces (75 ml) of pure white yogurt
- Two (2) teaspoons of maple syrup (optional, to taste) Ice cubes, to be served

88

1. Put the chopped kiwi and mango in the blender or blender together with the coconut milk.
2. Stir until large pieces of fruit begin to disappear, then add spirulina powder, yogurt, and maple syrup, if desired; keep fading until smooth.
3. Serve on ice and enjoy early!

31. BON APPÉTIT!

Whenever you sit down and savor every bite of your food, believe it or not, increasing your immunity. Many people think that digestion starts in the stomach, but the process begins in the mouth. Taking time to sit and chew food properly allows saliva to alkalize it (remember, bacteria prefer an acidic environment) and stimulates the production of essential digestive enzymes. The chewing process is a vital component of the digestive activities that occur in the mouth. It is inextricably linked to proper digestion and, therefore, to good health and immunity.

Taking time to enjoy food is not as easy as it seems: many of us rush meals and swallow more than we think. To get the maximum nutritional benefit that strengthens the immune system from food, you need to slow down and chew it thoroughly. So don't eat at your desk and don't try to eat something while running from one appointment to another. Set aside time to make sure that the food you eat is an adequate meal rather than just the fuel needed to get on board as quickly as possible.

The next time you eat or snack, focus on noting every single bite; what does it look like, smell and taste? Count to five between each bite or put the knife and fork between the bites. It doesn't take much time and effort to chew your food, and what you get in return is better digestion, better health, and more excellent immunity, as well as more enjoyment from your diet. Chewing and tasting food is important, but be sure to eat in a calm and peaceful environment. Avoid distractions that increase the likelihood of overeating or shoveling food without thinking about the mouth. Turn off the television and try not to read or work while eating.

CHAPTER FIVE
THE POWER OF WATER IN YOUR IMMUNE SYSTEM

We can only survive a week without water, while we can live up to six weeks without food. What are the vital links between our fluid intake and our immunity?

Water transports waste and toxins from our cells and the whole body. Some toxins are byproducts of our metabolism and immune function. Bacteria and other microbes produce some. Besides, toxins are introduced from natural or industrial sources through food, water, and air. Fortunately, water washes many of these toxins out of the body.

Water fills the systems that cleanse the body - blood and lymph, which are primarily water. Lymph is a liquid system loaded with antibodies (our immune artillery) and white blood cells. This system has been recognized for thousands of years as a source of purification: the Romans called it sap, which means "clear spring water."

This cleaning process is likely to help keep bacteria in balance. Although many of the bacteria in our body are useful we need to maintain this balance to stay healthy.

ARE YOU GETTING ENOUGH WATER?

Our bodies are about 70% water: ten to twelve gallons. We know that every cell in our body needs water to function and to provide nourishment and take away toxins. When these functions cannot be performed due to dehydration, several symptoms may occur.

- With 1% dehydration, most people are very thirsty, what is the body's warning sign that we need more fluids?

When we feel thirsty, we are already starting to dehydrate. People who are not naturally thirsty do not feel they are dehydrating.

- 2 to 5 percent of dehydration can cause dry mouth, redness of the skin, fatigue, headache, or impaired physical performance. We know that when the body becomes more dehydrated, there is less inclination towards exercise. Chronic low-grade dehydration can insinuate us. At this stage, signs of dehydration include:

1. Headache, which occurs when toxins begin to accumulate in the body
2. Poor digestion or constipation
3. Poor and darker colored urine
4. Extremely dry or itchy skin
5. Fatigue
6. Falls in concentration

- Dehydration of 6 to 8% can increase body temperature, respiratory rate, and pulse. We may have quite dramatic symptoms if we quickly dehydrate on a hot day or after intense exercise, experiencing:

1. Dizziness, fainting or nausea
2. Sudden weakness, fatigue or muscle cramps
3. Fatigue breathing from exertion

- Dehydration of 10 to 11 percent can cause muscle spasms or delirium. It can lead to poor blood circulation and even fail kidney function. Fifteen percent of dehydration can be fatal.

Check your water intake if you have experienced any of these symptoms and drink less than six glasses of water a day. So try gradually increasing the amount of water you drink until you have six to eight cups. So note if your health has improved.

Most of these symptoms are so common that any number of health conditions could cause them. This makes it challenging to determine what the underlying problem is. But getting enough liquid is an essential aspect of good health. Unfortunately, there is limited research on the link between immunity and dehydration. However, some people with chronic dehydration tend to be more often sick, afflicted with colds, flu, or other health problems.

WHY WATER IS IMPORTANT

In our bodies, water is how everything happens. Water carries nutrients and oxygen. It is essential for the digestion of proteins and fats and plays a vital role in effective energy production. Water also has particular functions: regulating body temperature by isolating from both heat and cold. Lubricates and softens the eyes, brain, and spinal cord, as well as joints and vital organs. Moistens and purifies our skin and the oxygen we breathe.

THE BODY IS MORE WATER
- Blood is made up of 83% water.
- The brain is made up of 75% water.
- Muscle is made up of 73% water.
- Fat is 25 percent water.
- The bone is made up of 22% water.

HOW MUCH WATER IS ENOUGH?
Americans are improving when it comes to drinking water: on average, about six cups of water per day, according to a 2000 survey. This represents an increase of 4.6 cups of water per day in 1998. However, many Americans report that having trouble. Frequent health problems, including fatigue and dizziness that can be caused by dehydration. A recent survey found that:
- Only a third relationship drinks eight or more glasses of water per day.
- Take three glasses of the drink or less per day.
- Nearly 10 percent don't drink water at all.

- We often hear that doctors recommend drinking six to eight glasses of water a day. A study in the Netherlands found that healthy older people looked at the drink, on average less than nine cups of water per day. Some of us need more, so determining your level is just as important. Like any other aspect of body chemistry, there is generally a personal balance point for each person.
- What is your ideal water consumption level? Consider your physical size, body type, the climate in which you live, and how active you are. It is also essential to know if further fluid intake is needed due to a special health condition (for example, the tendency to have kidney stones). On the other hand, if you are taking certain medications, it may be important not to drink too much liquid. Other determining factors include the amount of dehydrating drinks you drink, such as caffeine or alcohol.

WHAT TO DRINK

What are the best liquids to drink? According to the Rockefeller University Human Nutrition Center, water is the "best option for adequate hydration."

Springwater is one of the best options. Bottled waters also include glacial and mineral waters worldwide, including Canada, the French Alps, Fiji, Iceland, and Italy. Other good sources of water are bottled or tap water, which is well filtered, using a method such as carbon blocking or reverse osmosis filtration. Use bottled or filtered water in the kitchen to prepare herbal teas and dilute fresh fruit or vegetable juices.

What if the water tastes bad for you? Some people find that they don't like to drink water. In a recent consumer survey, 13% said they did not like the taste of water, and 12% said they preferred other drinks. For both problems, the answer may be to find a compatible type of water, such as imported water or light-flavored drinks. Adding a little aroma to the water can make drinking the right amount much more comfortable.

- Experiments to find the products you like the most.

- Enjoy the flavor of the wide variety of bottled waters and minerals.
- Flavor the water with one or two slices of lemon or lime.
- Add one sachet of herbal tea to the water at room temperature, hot or cold.
- Increase the nutrient content of water with a powder supplement such as Emergen-C or Ola Loa.
- Try slightly flavored waters like Fruit Water, which are now available for those who switch to water from fruit juices or sweeter drinks.
- Prepare fresh fruit juices (diluted approximately halfway with water).
- Try any of the light juices, such as AcquaBenessere or other products. Check the carbohydrate content on the label to make sure they don't contain the too much-added sweetener.
- According to traditional Chinese medicine, it is best to avoid frozen or icy drinks, due to the possible effect of extreme temperatures on the stomach.
- Enjoy hot or hot drinks such as herbal tea, green tea or chai; hot water with hot herbs like cinnamon and cardamom; ginger tea; lemon water; or vegetable broth.
- Hot water is considered a universal tonic throughout Asia and an effective remedy for many diseases. A healthy morning ritual begins by drinking something warm first, often merely hot water. This prepares the stomach, in the same way, that a hot shower revitalizes and makes the blood move. Drinking hot (but not boiling) water during the day is also considered very beneficial to health. It is believed to maintain or restore digestion.

INCREASE THE WATER INLET

Get enough water to drink. The most frequent reason provided by Americans for not drinking water is the lack of time, reported by 21% in a recent survey. Another 18 percent said having forgotten to drink water, not having good water, or being unable to rest benches. Many of these issues could be corrected, bringing bottled water or a favorite drink to work.

2. What happens if you are never thirsty? In a national survey, 8% said they were never thirsty. In another study, 10 percent reported never drinking water. The best way to deal with thirst is to drink water on time. Make sure it's a pleasant experience, something you can't wait to do. That means finding drinks you like and identifying times of day when you can drink something healthy. It can also involve a little extra logistics, such as buying a beautiful, leak-free ceramic mug for your desk or a cup holder for your car. Again, if there isn't a water cooler or filter at work, it also means bringing the bottled water you need every day.

3. Drink liquids at night. Going to bed isn't always the best time to drink water. Drinking water was mostly documented before 18:00. It can reduce the likelihood of late-night visits to the bathroom. Those who don't have this problem may find that the night is an excellent time to sit in another glass of water while reading, watching television or relaxing.

OTHER BEVERAGES

There are endless products on the market that taste and quench thirst. The key is to be aware of reading labels on drinks as well as on food. First, check the carbohydrate content for the amount of added sweeteners such as sugar, corn syrup, fructose, glucose, honey, maple syrup, fruit juice concentrate, or other additives that tend to promote weight gain when consumed in excess. Also, check the level of caffeine and other chemicals and food additives. If the drink dehydrates, such as coffee and alcohol, the solution is moderation.

1. Fruit juice. Bottled fruit juices are generally highly processed. The juice is cooked (pasteurized), bottled, and shipped, resulting in the inevitable destruction of vitamins and enzymes. What remains is the fruit sugar, fructose, which tastes good but has some drawbacks. A quarter of orange juice, for example, contains the extract of ten oranges. We hardly ever sit down to eat ten oranges, but we don't think of drinking a pint or even a liter of juice. Check the carbohydrate and sugar content with juice or soda so you know how sweet they are. An excellent way to avoid it is to eat fresh fruit instead of drinking juice.

2. Soft drinks. Carbonated drinks are rich in phosphoric acid, which contributes to osteoporosis, loss of calcium, and other minerals in the bones. They can also contain caffeine, artificial sweeteners, and other additives. Although artificial sweeteners prevent weight gain, research on most of these products has shown mixed results. As a gift, drinking soda with artificial sweeteners is probably not a problem. The problem becomes how often they are consumed: weekly, daily, or hourly?

In general, the craving for sweets can be reduced by drinking more water and other lighter drinks. Needs can also be minimized by taking buffered vitamin C or a chromium supplement. If you believe that your consumption of fruit, fruit juice, or soft drinks is excessive, make an effort to identify and eliminate the underlying cause through a resource such as Julia Ross's The Diet Cure.

DEHYDRATED DRINKS

We tend to forget that moisturizing and dehydrating drinks tend to cancel each other out. Moisturizing drinks are used to promote adequate water retention, the basis for a healthy function. Healthy drinks that keep the body hydrated include water, fruit juice, milk, and herbal teas. Caffeine-free carbonated drinks do not dehydrate but are often very sweetened.

Although Americans generally drink around eight servings of moisturizing drinks each day, they also have around five servings of dehydrating drinks per day. The most popular dehydrating drinks are coffee, tea, carbonated soft drinks containing caffeine, beer, wine, and other alcoholic beverages. Of these drinks, alcohol appears to be the most dehydrating. The drinks that dehydrate act as mild diuretics, increasing the production of urine and the loss of fluids from the body. They do not provide as much hydration to the body as moisturizing drinks. When we drink coffee, tea, soft drinks containing caffeine, and alcoholic drinks, we don't get the same moisturizing benefits as when we drink pure water.

COFFEE

In moderation, most food and drink is not a significant problem. A cup of coffee a day is not a problem for most people. If you're looking for a morning boost, try adding some form of protein to your breakfast (like a smoothie) and bring snacks that include some protein (like nuts) for later in the day. If coffee is just another drink for you, try switching to mineral or spring waters. If drinking coffee or tea is a social ritual, moderate your consumption by drinking herbal tea or green tea. When you want to get rid of the habit, you can try to gradually reduce your coffee intake by switching to lattes or cappuccinos.

ALCOHOLIC BEVERAGES

Research on alcohol consumption is mixed. Here, too, use discretion. Researchers recorded lower rates of heart disease among the French associated with red wine intake. In the United States, some studies have also found that moderate consumption of alcoholic beverages is related to greater relaxation and longer longevity. Although one or two glasses of wine a day have beneficial effects, they come at a price. It is well documented that alcoholic beverages have toxic effects on the liver and nervous system. They are linked to cancer and can be addictive. Since alcoholic beverages are also dehydrating, they should be subtracted from total water intake. Drink eight ounces of water for each alcoholic drink you drink.

WHEN WE NEED ADDITIONAL WATER

In some circumstances, we need to drink even more water than usual. To combat infections such as colds or flu, increasing water intake will help the lymphatic system eliminate germs and toxins. Drink more fluids if you have vomited or have diarrhea; Try something relaxing like mint, chamomile, or a combination of the two, like Sleepytime tea.

With some medications, it is essential not to drink too much water. With others, you may need to drink extra fluids. Find out which medications you are taking that may affect your hydration. Make sure you have all the facts.

Before and during exercise, drink liquids, and in particular, water, to lower body temperature, moderate cardiovascular stress, and improve performance. After intense training, it is vital to replace lost fluids.

WATER AND WEIGHTLOSS

For those seeking to lose weight, water is twice as beneficial as other drinks, as it does not contain the sweeteners, high calories, and carbohydrates found in soft drinks and sports drinks. To check the content of your drinks, simply read the carbohydrate and sugar information on the label of your favorite cooler. Beverages containing artificial sweeteners are not recommended. Water and soft drinks also tend to reduce food cravings; try it yourself.

REPLACEMENT OF FLUIDS DURING SPORTING EVENTS

1. Plain water is best for exercise that lasts an hour or less.
2. Don't depend on thirst. Drink before you are thirsty.
3. Drink water before a sporting event or physical activity. Take two cups of water two hours an event is successful.

4. Drink water during an event (1/4 to ¾ cup every ten to twenty minutes).

5. Take note of the weight before and after a sporting game or r intense training. After the game, replace the liquids with two cups of water for each pound lost.

The American College of Sports Medicine recommends that for training events lasting more than an hour, "Consider adding carbohydrates and electrolytes to a fluid replacement solution ... Containing 4 to 8 percent carbohydrates. "

PREGNANCY AND INGESTION OF WATER

Several common pregnancy disorders can be resolved by drinking enough water during pregnancy, including constipation, water retention, swelling, bladder infections, and hemorrhoids. Extreme dehydration can reduce the amount of amniotic fluid and may even be a factor in premature or difficult labor. An important way to minimize these pregnancy-related diseases is to drink lots of water. Water carries nutrients through the blood to the baby and is vital for maintaining good health during pregnancy. Experts recommend pregnant women to drink eight to ten eight-ounce glasses per day and one additional glass per hour of physical activity. Sufficient hydration can make the experience of pregnancy healthier and more pleasant for both mother and baby.

CHILDREN AND FLUIDS INTAKE

It is also important that children drink enough fluids. They are less equipped to handle high temperatures than adults because they have a lower sweating capacity. Therefore, in the heat, they need to drink even more water than adults. An additional benefit of giving children water or light drinks instead of too much juice or soda is that the potential for childhood obesity can be reduced.

When infants and young children are sick, frequent vomiting and severe diarrhea can quickly lead to dehydration. Weak rice water can be given to children with digestive problems. Fluid replacement is best done with water that contains electrolytes (minerals, a little salt, and a little sweetener) to maintain the correct balance of fluids. Electrolytes can be purchased as products like Gatorade or small packets of electrolyte minerals in the health food store. You can also make an electrolytic solution at home:

- 1 liter of drinking water or boiled water
- 2 tbsp. Honey or sugar
- ¼ tsp. Sea salt or table salt
- ¼ tsp. baking soda (baking soda)
- Optional: ½ cup of orange juice can be added to increase the potassium content.

MAKE THE WATER PRETTY DRINKING

Over time, encourage your child to try various soft drinks that we describe here. For thirsty children, these drinks seem to make the most significant difference if they drink enough fluids daily. Good options include:

1. Fresh juice or half juice and half spring water
2. Light bottled drinks such as fruit water or light juices
3. Simple homemade soups
4. Tasty and nutritious blending drinks
5. Herbal tea without caffeine
6. Light soy drinks

- Make sure you don't overdo your child's carbohydrate intake with too much fruit, fruit juice, sweet vegetables like carrots, or many sweeteners that are also found in seemingly nutritious products. Monitor your carbohydrate intake by reading the labels.
- Encourage your child to get into the habit of drinking water or something light in the morning and, if possible, an hour before breakfast and dinner.
- Use fresh and colorful mugs, bottles, and straws to spark your interest in drinking more.
- On hot days, keep the water cold but not cold.

- When you shop, you make the right decisions. Don't fill the refrigerator with too many tempting drinks full of sugar and caffeine that could derail your efforts.
- Be a good example by drinking lots of water and liquids too!

DEHYDRATION AND AGING

As we age, our thirst decreases. Perhaps consequently, dehydration, which can sometimes be fatal, is one of the most frequent causes of hospitalization in people over the age of sixty-five. Aging is also associated with lower levels of total body fluids, reduced fitness, and reduced kidney function, which can contribute to dehydration. You can compensate for the subtle loss of function as part of the natural aging process by drinking extra fluids to keep the body detoxified. Age can be considered a fountain of youth.

HOW IMPORTANT IS WATER FOR OUR HEALTH?

Although we don't have extensive research yet, we have to draw definite conclusions; doctors have noticed a link between drinking enough water and good health. Why haven't we heard more about the importance of drinking water? Research is expensive. Like the air we breathe, water cannot be patented. As a result, lifestyle factors tend to be less studied.

Conditions that can be improved by drinking enough water include:

- Hyperacidity
- Constipation
- Mild mood swings
- Kidney stones. Anyone with a history of kidney stones can benefit from adequate water intake, as water dissolves calcium in the urine, reducing the risk of stone formation. Among doctors, urologists are likely to enhance the virtues of water.
- Urinary tract infections. For men and women, this can be avoided by drinking enough water.

You can see the effects of drinking water on your health. Make sure to proceed gradually. Consider taking electrolyte capsules if your water intake exceeds eight cups a day.

Contact your doctor for advice on what's right for you. Enjoy!

CHAPTER SIX
PREVENTION OF CHRONIC AND
AUTOIMMUNE DISEASES

Driving a healthy way of life by settling on sound decisions can bring about a more extended, progressively free, and more joyful life. There are many things that you can do to help carry on with a good life and forestall ceaseless disease and disease. Six suggested healthy living methodologies include:

- Physical Activity
- Good dieting
- Living Smoke-Free
- Restricting Alcohol Intake
- Deal with Your Stress
- Getting Screened for Cancer
- Get Enough Sleep
- Physical Activity: Be dynamic. Get going!

Being dynamic can add many advantages to your life. Research shows that being physically active for 150 minutes out of every week can reduce the danger of heart illness, stroke, hypertension, specific kinds of disease, type 2 diabetes, osteoporosis, and overweight. Physical activity is likewise connected with better emotional wellness, stress help, and feeling good.

To accomplish medical advantages and improve useful capacities, the Canadian Physical Activity Guidelines suggest that grown-ups, ages 18 to 64 years, amass 150 minutes of moderate-to-enthusiastic vigorous movement every week, in episodes of 10 minutes or more. You ought to likewise attempt to join quality preparing and adaptability into your week by week schedule.

Put the tablet down, turn off the TV, and get dynamic! Being active doesn't need to be desolate or exhausting. Bring a companion and discover an activity that you appreciate. You can even incorporate physical activity with your day by day schedule for more prominent comfort. Being truly dynamic is likewise connected with better psychological wellness and stress alleviation.

Good dieting: You are what you eat.

Your body is a stunning machine, yet it needs healthy fuel to perform at its best. An eating diet that continually takes care of the body fried, high-fat, salty junk food resembles emptying bacon oil into your vehicle's gas tank – it will simply obstruct the motor and keep it from working appropriately.

Canada's Food Guide suggests eating a larger number of vegetables and natural products than some other nutritional category. In case you're a grown-up somewhere in the range of 19 and 50 years old, Canada's Food Guide suggests that females eat 7-8 servings of vegetables and products of the soil eat 8-10 servings.

8 servings may appear to be a ton; however, it truly isn't. For instance, a ½ cup of fresh, frozen, or canned vegetables and natural products consider 1 serving. 1 cup of raw verdant vegetables, for example, salad, is another serving. For the day, those servings can include quicker than you know it!

Did you realize that you should drink 8 glasses of water every day? Your body is made generally out of the water, so you need to ensure you are hydrated for ideal health. Attempt to evade sweet beverages with void calories and drink water.

In our bustling lives and surged condition, it is difficult to depend on cheap food or pre-made bites. Here are a few hints to assist you with keeping up healthy adjusted eating diets:

- Keep a water bottle with you, so you drink water and not squeeze or pop.
- Keep healthy snacks close by grinding away (for example, carrot sticks, unsalted nuts, oranges, and so forth.)
- Put together a lunch for school and work.
- Plan your week by week menu
- Live Smoke-Free

The absolute best thing that you can do to prevent chronic disease and avoid premature death is to live without smoke.

Smoking is a realized hazard factor for building up a few ceaseless illnesses, for example, cardiovascular disease and a few kinds of diseases. Know that it is never past the point where it is possible to stop. Your body begins to mend itself inside long stretches of stopping. Inside 8 hours, your carbon monoxide levels in your blood drop and oxygen levels rise. Following 2 days, your feeling of smell and taste begin to improve. Between about fourteen days and 3 months, you will think that it's simpler to inhale because your lungs are working better. If you remain smoke-free for a year, your risk of a smoking-related respiratory failure is sliced down the middle.

Smoking isn't a propensity; rather, it is a dependence on nicotine – one of the world's most remarkable medications. If you or somebody you know is attempting to stop smoking, there is help accessible. Research shows that around 70% of individuals who smoke have pondered stopping or need to stop.

With an end goal to help a healthy environment for our patients, families, staff, and volunteers, our Hospital's grounds are 100% without smoke.

Breaking point Your Alcohol Intake

Sound living methods everything with some restraint – and that incorporates drinking liquor. Late reports show that drinking beyond what the suggested measure of liquor can build your danger of liver sickness, cardiovascular illness, and a few sorts of cancer.

Cancer anticipation rules suggest that, whenever expended, liquor ought to be constrained to 1 beverage for ladies and 2 beverages for men every day. If you decide to drink, consider these more secure drinking tips:

- Set cutoff points for yourself and stick to them.
- Drink gradually. Have close to 2 beverages in any 3 hours.
- For each drink of liquor, have one non-mixed beverage.
- Eat previously and keeping in mind that you are drinking.

- Continuously think about your age, body weight, and health programs that may recommend lower limits.
- While drinking may give medical advantages to specific meetings of individuals, don't begin to drink or increment your drinking for medical advantages.

Deal with Your Stress: Relax. Discover balance.

We live in a quick-paced, occupied world, and at times, we become involved with the movements of everyday life and stresses. Roughly 58% of Canadians report 'over-burden' because of the weights related to work, home life, and extracurricular exercises.

Set aside a few minutes for yourself to unwind or do the things you appreciate. Discover the parity in your life between work, life, and the entirety of your other everyday organizations in the middle of – including getting enough rest! Make it your need to discover a work-life balance. Snap here for certain tips on the best way to help discover balance.

Get Screened for Cancer!

Cancer screening can discover tumors before when they are simpler to treat.

Get a good night's rest.

In some cases, we overlook how significant getting enough rest is, yet it is significant for ideal health. Grown-ups should mean to get 7 to 9 hours of rest each night Click here for some sound rest tips.

Constant Disease Prevention Messages:

- Anideal approach to battle constant sickness and disease is to forestall it.
- Grown-ups, ages 18 to 64, ought to collect 150 minutes of activity every week.
- Before beginning an activity program, you should converse with your PCP.
- Being dynamic at any rate, 150 minutes out of each week can reduce the danger of interminable disease and unexpected passing.

- Physical movement can prompt improved wellness, quality, and emotional wellness.
- Eat at any rate one dark green and one orange vegetable every day.
- Have vegetables and natural products more regularly than juice.
- Select lean meats and cut back obvious excess from meats.
- A solitary cigarette contains more than 4,000 chemicals.
- The absolute best thing you can accomplish for your health is to live without smoke.
- The vast majority who smoke have contemplated stopping or need to stop.
- Smoking isn't a propensity; it is a dependence on nicotine.
- Discover your work-life balance.
- Get screened for cancer!
- Grown-ups ought to get 7 to 9 hours of rest each night.

CHAPTER SEVEN
HOW TO IMPROVE YOUR SLEEP AND BOOST ENERGY

HOW MUCH DO YOU NEED?

Are you sleepy? There is total agreement that sleep is vital for your immunity. However, we also know that sleep requirements are very individual and vary significantly from person to person. Therefore, to stay as healthy as possible, we want to find our ideal balance between sleep, rest, and activity.

For anyone with problems with a disease, getting what you need is even more critical. Quality sleep has several beneficial effects. It offers the body the opportunity to rest and repair itself. Also, when we are awake and active for a shorter period, the body accumulates less metabolic toxins. Now, studies by the National Institutes of Health provide compelling evidence that the immune system is not fully activated during at least nine and a half hours of sleep or more.

If you want to increase your immune response, whether you're battling a sudden cold or struggling with a long-term illness, try to lengthen the hours you sleep until you wake up naturally, refreshed. You may need a maximum of twenty-four hours of bed rest and as much sleep as possible to recover if you are sick.

IS DREAM A DEMAND FOR LIFE OR DEATH?

Accidents such as the Exxon Valdez oil spill and the Chernobyl and Three Mile Island nuclear accidents have been linked to human errors caused by lack of sleep. At least 100,000 road accidents are said to be caused by drowsiness or fatigue each year, resulting in deaths for over 1,500 Americans and 71,000 others injured. In a recent National Sleep Foundation survey, about one in five drivers reported falling asleep behind the wheel in the past year. Sleep loss is a problem that affects most of us. Most Americans report not getting enough sleep:

- Adults. Seven out of ten say they have frequent sleep problems.
- Teenagers. Nearly nine out of ten say they need more sleep.
- Children. More than two out of five have difficulty falling asleep or feeling fatigued.

We all know that sleep is essential, but it is often one of the first things we are willing to sacrifice for other priorities. Most of us feel we don't have enough rest. But just enough? In the 1950s, the American Cancer Society conducted an extensive investigation into the effect of lifestyle on health. Volunteers have interviewed more than 1 million Americans in every county and parish in the United States. UU. Participants were asked about their exercise, nutrition, smoking, sleep, and other health habits.

Seven years later, the survey was repeated. The pollsters collected data on all the original participants who died after the first survey. The information was analyzed and re-analyzed to determine the most important lifestyle factors for health and survival. Sleep loss was the factor most associated with mortality.

The lowest mortality rates were for survey respondents who said they averaged eight hours of sleep per night. Studies have since had similar results: eight hours of sleep appear to be related to good health. The highest mortality rate at all ages was for those with an average of four hours or less of sleep per night. A large body of animal research on sleep deprivation confirms the adverse health effects of sleep loss.

Currently, however, over two-thirds of Americans report not sleeping eight hours a night.

SLEEVELESS IN AMERICA

In a recent national survey, seven out of ten Americans say they have frequent sleep problems. However, most have not been diagnosed by a doctor. More than eight out of ten say they will sleep more if they knew they could be healthier. The survey found that one in five adults are so sleepy during the day that it interferes with daily activities a few days a week or more.

- The American US workforce work for longer hours. Americans work harder and sleepless. He already works more hours than workers in any industrialized nation in the world, with an average of forty-six hours a week in the workplace. More than one-third of the workforce works for more than fifty hours a week. As a result, many of us feel pressured and stressed.
- Stress. Sleep can also be lost due to stress, reflected in symptoms such as worry, fatigue, physical tension, depression, or anxiety.
- Health problems. Perhaps the most crucial physical problem that interferes with sleep quality is chronic pain, from conditions such as injury, arthritis, ulcers, or headaches. Obstructive sleep apnea, a condition in which breathing is partially obstructed during sleep, is now recognized as more common than previously thought. The diagnosis of sleep apnea often requires expert evaluation in a sleep clinic.
- Nutritional deficiencies. For example, some people with insomnia appear to have a higher calcium requirement, corrected by merely taking a calcium and magnesium supplement overnight.

Overall, according to a national survey, about half of the population suffers from insomnia. Over half of the respondents reported feeling so sleepy at work that they compromised the quality of their work. Signs of sleep loss in adults include:

- Reduced immunity
- Daytime sleepiness
- Less interest in the exercise.
- Mood swings, depression, anxiety, and irritability.
- Increased stress
- Memory impaired

- Reduced ability to handle complex tasks or solve problems
- Reduced coordination
- Disorientation
- Increased risk of road accidents.

SLEEP LOSS AND TEENAGERS

We never really get used to inadequate sleep. Dr. William Dement, director of the Stanford Center for Sleep Disorders and founder of the sleep medicine industry, suggests that most people accumulate a sleep deficit and suffer the consequences. For teenagers, these include the decline in cognitive functioning and disease resistance, behavioral abnormalities, and, in extreme cases, traffic accidents caused by falling asleep while driving.

The best available data on the relationship between adolescent sleep and academic achievement comes from studies in Rhode Island and Minnesota. In 1998, Rhode Island researchers interviewed 3,000 high school students to document their sleep deficit and link it to daytime functioning and school performance. In the survey, 87 percent of students reported needing more sleep. Older teens slept less than younger teens. The research proofs that only 5 percent of parents decided to go to sleep in school evening. Teenagers with a lack of sleep seem to have symptoms similar to adults: fatigue, a bad mood, and lack of alertness. Also, the following may occur:
- Lack of motivation
- Behavioral anomalies
- Hyperactivity

The study did not show a direct relationship between sleep patterns and school grades. However, she found that students who described themselves as "struggling or failing at school" reported fewer hours of sleep, irregular hours, and later bedtime than students who performed well. Why wasn't there a more direct link between grades and sleep loss? The accumulation of sleep debt tends to affect long-term performance.

A Minnesota school board experimented with offering students more opportunities to recover sleep by opening schools an hour later. After the first year, 57% of teachers reported that students were more alert during the early two periods of the day. A previous study in Minnesota has received even more positive reviews.

LOSS OF CHILDREN SLEEP AND SCHOOL

Even younger children have sleep problems. In a survey conducted by parents in Washington, DC, about 11% reported that their baby had recently had a sleep disorder that had lasted more than two weeks. And over 20 percent of parents said their son took too long to fall asleep, snore or tire during the day at least once a week.

For young people, eight hours of sleep may not be enough; it may take eight to nine hours of sleep per night or more. The signs that children have difficulty sleeping include all the symptoms observed in adults. Additional indications that can be seen in children include:
- Difficulty falling asleep.
- Waking up frequently during the night or insomnia.
- Speak during sleep or nightmares.
- Difficulty breathing properly
- Bedwetting
- Tighten or clamp the teeth.

QUALITY SLEEP

When it comes to sleep, quality seems to be as important as quantity. A recent Finnish study found parallels between proper sleep and good health. The researchers looked at the sleep quality and health status of 1,600 Finnish adults. The survey showed that men with poor quality sleep were six times more likely to have health problems. Women who slept poorly were more than three times more likely to have health problems.

THE EFFECT OF SLEEP LOSS

Does it matter when we lose some sleep? For more than ten years, animal and human studies have been conducted to answer this question. When studying a lack of sleep, it is described in

112

terms of sleep debt, mainly sleep loss. Typically, animal or human subjects are kept awake for a specified period. Then their blood is measured to determine levels of chemical markers such as T cells. The results obtained from animal studies can be applied to humans because sleep functions, body chemistry, and the immune system are quite similar in mammals. Here is a summary of what researchers have found that will help you decide how important sleep is.

LOST FIVE HOURS OF SLEEP IN A SINGLE NIGHT

A study at the University of California, San Diego, involved young, healthy volunteers. Losing just five hours of sleep a night has been found to depress your natural immune responses. There has been a 30 percent reduction in T cells that fight infections, natural killer cells. An essential immune enhancer, the anticancer interleukin known as IL-2, was also depressed. After a night of sleep recovery, T cell activity returned to its original level, but interleukin levels remained depressed. These results suggest the importance of sleep in maintaining immunity and show "that even moderate sleep disturbance causes a reduction in natural immune responses."

LOST FOUR HOURS TO STAY ONE NIGHT, FOR SIX NIGHTS

A study published in The Lancet indicates how sleep loss can affect metabolism. University of Chicago researchers studied physical changes in eleven young people who slept only four hours a night, six nights in a row. They found that lack of sleep seemed to trigger a temporary condition that resembled diabetes, interfering with hormone production, and its ability to metabolize starches and sugars. In response to these and other similar results, some researchers suggest that sleeping more helps the body maintain excess weight.

FIVE DAYS WITHOUT SLEEP

Research on short sleep deficits has shown a variety of effects. In some studies, sleep-deprived animals have shown a reduction in protective antibody levels. A decrease in antibody levels was also found in a Norwegian survey that monitored men in military training who had been sleepless for about five days. The most dramatic declines were in antibodies that respond to immediate infection, IgM, which decreased by 35 percent. White blood cell counts also reduced by 30 to 50 percent. To date, an inconsistent picture emerges from short-term sleep deficit studies. Some research has reported low levels of immunity. In contrast, others have found that specific aspects of the immune response have increased after short-term sleep loss. However, increases in anti-stress hormone levels suggest that sleep loss can cause metabolic stress.

DO NOT SLEEP FOR FORTY DAYS

The biggest concern is the evidence found in long-term sleep loss studies. Forty-day sleep deprivation proved fatal for animals in research conducted at the National Institute of Mental Health. Autopsies have found massive levels of bacteria in the blood and lymph nodes of animals. Dr. Carol Everson and her colleagues concluded that prolonged sleep deprivation appears to cause "a collapse of the host's defense against harmful bacteria."

Signs and symptoms resulting from long-term sleep deprivation included weakened appearance, skin lesions, burnout syndrome, increased energy expenditure, decreased body temperature during the later stages of denial, and increased hormone levels. Four other essential anomalies were also detected:
* Malnutrition
* Decreased mental function.
* Low thyroid levels
* Reduction of resistance to infections.

Immune activity during sleep appears to maintain balance within the body. It seems that one of the essential functions of sleep is to provide the body with time to reduce the levels of bacteria in the system. A wide range of yeasts and bacteria usually is present in the digestive tract, many of which are useful. As long as your levels remain in balance, they are not a problem.

Therefore, sleeping seems to provide an opportunity for some sort of internal cleansing.

The amount of sleep required is unique for each of us. Research confirms this and also suggests that there is a genetic basis for our sleep needs. At the University of Texas, researchers monitored behavior and brain waves in two types of rats. They discovered a constant difference in sleep patterns from one species to another. Animal studies at the University of Geneva in Switzerland also found consistent variations. They reported that the study result "strongly suggests the presence of a gene with a significant effect" on the amount of sleep required. This genetic difference has also been confirmed in research at the Helioski University in Finland.

We never get used to it without sleeping. But we all know from personal experience that the body recovers from sleep loss. What do you need to recover from sleep debt? Animals suffering from sleep loss were allowed to sleep as much as they wanted in the second phase of a study at the University of Chicago. Over fifteen days, most animals showed a complete or almost complete reversal of symptoms, including improvements in their appearance and energy. They restored the balance of the thyroid and stress hormones. The researchers reported that "the salient features of sleep recovery ... were immediate." In some animals, the recovery process took longer. This is another example of individual variation.

GOOD SLEEP AT NIGHT

Supporting the immune system through sleep may require a change in lifestyle. It could mean letting go of certain pleasures or exchanging one desire for another. Instead of staying awake to watch your favorite show, you may want to record the show. Instead, take a hot shower or a lush bath and rest for a long, delicious sleep.

REMEDIES FOR SLEEPING

If you wish to reset your internal clock by promoting previous sleep patterns, there are a few remedies that can come in handy. Before using a herbal or nutritional remedy, and if you have a health condition or are taking any medications, be sure to consult your doctor appropriately. The safest approach is to start with minimal doses, for example taking only one capsule a day for the first three days. When it is clear that the remedy conforms to your system, gradually increase it to the recommended dose. Avoid making other changes during that time, so if there is a problem, the cause is apparent.

NAPPING

Does a nap make up for lost sleep at night? There is also good evidence that naps are useful according to several studies, including those conducted at Henry Ford Hospital in Detroit. The rest has been found "clearly useful for someone who usually sleeps but cannot sleep enough at night... We don't understand the underlying neurobiology, but sleep time is cumulative. A nap of two or four hours before [stay] awake all night, provides additional attention the next day. " NASA research has found similar results. However, it is essential not to take a nap too close to bedtime, as it may interrupt your necessary sleep.

INSOMNIA

A doctor or sleep expert best addresses insomnia that continues for more than three months. There are now sleeping centers located in the United States. The USA, listed in The Promise of Sleep, by Dr. William Dement.

REST AND SLEEP

There is a big difference between resting in bed and sleeping. Sleep that allows for a deeper state of rest is particularly important, as it offers the opportunity to bring metabolic recovery into the body to a level that does not seem to occur only through rest. We know from recent research that a prolonged period of sleep is required for the immune system to be compromised entirely, which is why we typically sleep much longer when we are sick. Research also suggests that deep sleep allows for more excellent antibody production.

SLEEP AND IMMUNITY

Experience and common sense suggest that rest is helpful when we are sick. We also see this wisdom in animals that can sleep up to a week when they are ill or injured. From a scientific point of view, research has shown the essential role of sleep in promoting immunity. Given all these tests, the biggest challenge may simply be to act on that wisdom. This means finding ways to adapt to sleep to our busy lives. Sweet dreams.

IN SHORT:

- For young people, the amount of sleep needed appears to be more than eight hours: eight and a half, nine or more hours per night.
- According to NIH research, when we are sick, we need a maximum of nine and a half hours of sleep per night or more.
- An excellent way to find out how much sleep you need to go to bed at the same time every night and see what time you naturally wake up without an alarm clock.
- What is the best sleep cycle? Depending on your makeup, you may also have to go to bed early to wake up refreshed. So, if you still wake up feeling tired after a night of sleep, go to bed gradually before being naturally well-rested. You may even find yourself a little disoriented for a few days as your body adjusts to its new sleep schedule.
- It may take up to two weeks to regain sleep in case of sleep deficiency.

CHAPTER EIGHT
HEALTHY LIFESTYLE/SPORTS TO AUGMENT YOUR BODY DEFENSES

THE LINK BETWEEN PHYSICAL ACTIVITIES AND IMMUNITY DEFENSES

Many of us have transformed the old aphorism that exercise is good for us into a kind of fur shirt. We believe that if we don't exercise a lot, that is, a lot of sweat and pain, we won't get any benefit. Nothing is further from the truth. From an immune system point of view, moderate exercise is ideal, which means that walking four times a week will increase the immune system's function and protect it from infections, cancer, and heart disease.

However, exercise presents a stimulating paradox when considered solely in terms of benefits for the immune system. On the one hand, people live longer and enjoy better health when exercising regularly and moderately. However, exercise is a stressful factor in the body, especially the immune system. Heavy exercise depresses some immune cell counts, at least temporarily. Furthermore, very stressful long-term training programs, such as competitive long-distance running, resulting in consistently lower immunity, at least for some immune factors.

Therefore, contrary to what many believe, there is excessive exercise. And like many other examples of "overdoing something good," excessive exercise can weaken the immune response to pathogens. These revelations teach us, once again, that balance is crucial for good health.

Interestingly, the effect of exercise on the immune system largely depends on the degree of effort and almost nothing on time spent exercising. For example, thirty seconds of intense exercise causes changes in the relative number of white blood cells in the blood. In contrast, one hour of gentle exercise has no measurable effect on these cells. Besides, the changes observed after thirty minutes of moderate exercise are the same as those found after two hours of the same level of training.

Despite the fact that exercise has been studied so thoroughly, especially its impact on the cardiovascular system, many remain to be learned about what exercise functions for the immune system's funtion. In general, people who exercise moderately live longer and have lower rates of cancer and cardiovascular disease. Most of these benefits may be related to the immune system. For example, moderate exercise increases the function of macrophages. These cells play a crucial role in creating atherosclerosis and heart disease. Recognizing this effect, some scientists have speculated that the benefits of exercise for macrophage cells may represent independent protection against heart disease and the known benefits of exercise for heart function, circulation, and respiration.

However, this and other questions have not yet been answered. What we do know is that moderate exercise has the best impact on the immune system.

THE IMMUNE SYSTEM AND THE EXERCISE: SOME GOOD NEWS, SOME BAD

FIRST GOOD NEWS

The effects of exercise on the immune system that has been most extensively studied are changes in the number and type of white blood cells, the proliferation capacity of lymphocytes, and the ability of natural killer cells to destroy target cells. In general, the number of all major classes of white blood cell granulocytes, natural killer cells, monocytes (the current form of macrophages), and lymphocytes increases during exercise, especially if the exercise has not been very strenuous.

MACROPHAGES

Moderate exercise makes macrophages swallow bacteria, viruses, and cancer cells more aggressively. It also causes macrophages to produce more health-promoting cytokines, including interleukin-1 (which causes inflammation), interleukin-6 (which is also pro-inflammatory), and tumor necrosis factor (which kills cancer cells and tumors).

Overall, research shows that macrophages respond to exercise in the same way they react to infections. In essence, they become more alert and aggressive toward possible health threats. Macrophages become particularly active in inflammation area, which can be one of the reasons why exercise is associated with lower rates of cancer. Some studies have shown that macrophages enter muscle tissue and attack antigens after use.

GRANULOCYTES

After a period of moderate exercise, granulocytes are more aggressive in the consumption and destruction of antigens. They also show a marked improvement in their ability to target areas of the body where they may be needed and destroy foreign or invasive bacteria or viruses.

NATURAL KILLER CELLS

Like macrophages and granulocytes, natural killer cells are more aggressive and more numerous after moderate exercise. The exercise appears to correctly promote the ability of natural killer cells to destroy tumors. This effect also occurs in older women who continuously start and maintain training programs.

Exercise-induced immune changes tend to be short-lived. Most increases or decreases in immune cells return to normal within fifteen minutes or two hours after exercise, although some last a day or longer.

BAD NEWS NOW

However, the proliferation ability of lymphocytes is suppressed after exercise. However, this weakening of immunity appears to be short-lived and returns to normal in an hour or two. However, when T cells become slow, their ability to produce cytokines, such as interleukin-2, is reduced. This means that B cells are also less sensitive to antigens, as they depend on CD4 cells to command them to produce antibodies.

The reduced immune response after exercise seems to be more influential among competitive athletes who participate in very demanding training regimens.

ON TRAINING AND IMMUNITY RESPONSE

Exercise alters the blood levels of some stress hormones, such as cortisol, epinephrine, and beta-endorphin. The quantity and types of hormones produced vary according to the kind of exercise and degree of difficulty. The more intense the workout, the more these stress hormones are created. Stress hormones, as we will see in chapter 9, tend to weaken the immune response.

One of the great benefits of exercise is that it pumps more oxygen into the blood, but there is also a dark side to the advantage here. As the cells breathe or breathe, they produce more oxidants, which split the molecules and form free radicals. This, in turn, increases the demand for some antioxidants in the cells and bloodstream, especially for glutathione. The combination of hormonal changes, high oxidants, and increased demand for antioxidants creates strains on the immune system, which, for those on a poor diet, can weaken overall immunity.

There is a well-known relationship between overtraining in athletes and increased susceptibility to infections. In studies that compared the immune responses of highly trained athletes with those of the control populations, the athletes were losers. Blood lymphocyte levels, immunoglobulin levels in blood and saliva, and the ratio of CD4 cells to CD8 cells were lower in athletes than in controls. The natural activity of killer cells was also more moderate in athletes.

The adverse effects of excessive exercise are likely to be a combination of psychological and physical stress, along with a depletion of antioxidants in the bloodstream. As the German national field hockey team prepared for the 1988 Olympics, the combination of intense exercise during training and the psychological stress of approaching the competition led to considerable depressions in the players' immune system. Some players had a CD4 cell count typical of AIDS patients.

The improved nutrition of athletes seems to compensate for at least some of the adverse effects of overtraining. One study showed that marathon runners who received vitamin C after a race had lower rates of respiratory infections than those who didn't receive the vitamin, suggesting that replacing antioxidants helps mitigate the adverse effects of exercise. Other studies have supported the conclusion that, in addition to following a highly nutritious diet, competitive athletes who undergo intense training should take antioxidants after intense exercise.

THE EFFECTS OF THE EXERCISE ON DISEASE

CANCER

Exercise seems to offer women significant protection against breast cancer. A recent study showed that use reduced breast cancer risk in Caucasian women in their forties and younger, especially those who had children. Women who exercised at least forty-eight minutes a week on average were less likely to develop cancer than those who exercised less or none. Maximum protection was observed in those who exercised more, more than 3.8 hours per week.

In general, there is a lower incidence of some cancers in those who exercise regularly than in those who do not.

ASTHMA AND ALLERGIES

For those with asthma and allergies, the best form of exercise seems to be yoga. Intense exercise, on the other hand, can cause problems.

Many studies indicate that exercise can trigger an asthmatic episode and allergic reactions. The tendency to provoke such results may be due to the production of catecholamines (norepinephrine and epinephrine, which create excitement) during exercise.

Yoga seems to be an exception to this as it does not cause asthmatic or allergic reactions. Also, at least one study has shown that yoga has improved lung function and reduced the need for medications for young asthmatics.

ARTHRITIS

According to research in which people with arthritis have been followed for four years, there are no adverse effects, such as joint destruction, from exercise for arthritis patients. A routine exercise program is vital for people with rheumatoid arthritis to increase cardiovascular strength, muscle endurance, and overall strength.

A study examining the effects of the Asian tai chi chuan exercise showed that martial art of dance did not cause any harmful effects and was safe for people with rheumatoid arthritis.

CROHN'S DISEASE

Exercise reduces the incidence of Crohn's disease, a form of inflammatory bowel disease. Those who exercise regularly have fewer outbreaks of the disease than those who do not.

CHRONIC FATIGUE SYNDROME

People with chronic fatigue syndrome who exercise moderately for thirty minutes a day show reduced fatigue, confusion, and depression.

INFECTIONS

Those who exercise moderately have the least number of diseases, while those who train intensely, such as marathon runners, appear to have higher infection rates, especially after a competitive event.

STRESS AND EMOTIONAL PROBLEMS

Exercise increases mood and relieves stress and depression. By elevating mood and increasing positive feelings about yourself and life in general, exercise indirectly improves the immune system's function.

A study published in Postgraduate Medicine (July 1990) reported that people who had previously suffered from depression and other emotional problems experienced reductions in stress and anxiety and experienced fewer bouts of depression after starting to exercise. Her ability to cope with stress is also increased with regular exercise. When stressful situations occurred, they did not give in to self-criticism and other types of negative thoughts. These mental habits existed before starting the exercise. The researchers also found that constant exercise seemed to trigger a kind of emotional transformation. The researchers reported feeling healthier, more loving, brighter, and much more positive than life.

These effects are not merely superficial mood swings, but alterations in brain chemistry. The brain starts producing beta-endorphins after only twenty minutes of operation. Chronic depression has also been alleviated with constant exercise.

When it comes to relieving stress and increasing mood, aerobic exercise appears to have a more significant impact than anaerobic activities, such as weight training. When the psychological effects of aerobic exercise were compared to those of weight training and without exercise, the researchers found that aerobic exercise had the most significant impact on mood and sense of well-being.

EXERCISE, AGING, AND LONGEVITY

A study in older women showed that upper respiratory tract infections were lower in those who exercised regularly, and particularly low among women who had calisthenics periodically. Respiratory diseases were highest among those who did not exercise. Women whose only exercise was walking also benefited from fewer respiratory infections; however, they did not have a low infection rate like those whose programs included regular calisthenics.

Not surprisingly, these immune improvements affect the quality of life, as people of any age who exercise regularly experience lower rates of chronic and degenerative diseases. Besides, studies have shown that colds, bacterial infections, and flu viruses don't last long in people who exercise regularly.

Scientists from the Aerobics Research Institute and Cooper Clinic in Dallas studied a group of 13,344 men and women for over eight years to determine the effect, if any, on longevity. Scientists measured subjects' fitness levels directly by walking people on a treadmill, rather than merely filling out questionnaires. The participant that participated in the study were divided into five groups, based on how fitness they are. Fitness groups varied from those who lived a sedentary lifestyle to well-conditioned athletes. As expected, those who were most sedentary died as soon as possible.

However, scientists were surprised to find that the most prominent health benefits came from those who simply walked and walked half an hour a day, three or four times a week. This small amount of exercise reduces the risk of heart attack or cancer by more than half.

Other research has confirmed these results. A study published in the New England Journal of Medicine (February 25, 1993) found that men who play vigorous sports between the ages of forty-five and fifty-four live on average ten months longer than those who remain sedentary.

HOW MUCH EXERCISE DO YOU NEED?

The overall impact of exercise on the immune system depends mostly on the degree of effort and almost nothing on time spent exercising. The changes observed after thirty minutes of moderate exercise are the same as those found after two hours from the same exercise once the rhythm is reached, the body tends to adapt and maintain its balance.

To benefit from an aerobic program, you need to exercise for at least twenty minutes a day, three or four days a week. According to the American College of Sports Medicine, you should train at a rate that increases your heart rate from 60 to 90 percent of your maximum. To avoid immunity that suppresses the effects of overtraining, 80% of the maximum is a cautious goal.

To determine your maximum heart rate, subtract your age from 220. The heart rate of 50 years and older people is a maximum of 170. To benefit from a training session, a 50-year-old child must reach a heart rate of 102 to 136 beats per minute and keep it there for 20 minutes.

Before starting your workout, warm up by doing ten minutes of stretching exercises. Starting a slower pace than your optimal speed and gradually increase your training speed is the way to go if you choose to work. This will prepare your heart, respiratory system, and muscles for your training. When you are finished exercising, stretch again slightly from five to ten minutes to cool down.

Very important: before starting the exercise, ask your doctors to do a complete checkup. Do not practice competitive sports if you are not in shape and have not trained for a while. People forget about themselves in the heat of competition and try too hard, which sometimes leads to heart attacks. Start slowly and move towards a more demanding program.

AN EXERCISE PROGRAM FOR THE PROMOTION OF IMMUNITY

1. Choose a time during the day when you can train and stick to that moment. Most people like to teach in the morning. You only need twenty or thirty minutes, during which you can walk the block at least once and, more than once, your fitness improves.
2. Exercise during the day. Go up the stairs instead of taking the elevator. Walk for lunch instead of taking a taxi. Take a walk after lunch.
3. Fun is the key. Choose an activity or sport that you like to do and become useful. Popular exercises include walking, mountain biking, tennis, swimming, water aerobics, and home weight training.
4. Join the club. Signing up for a YMCA, YWCA, or spa is a great way to train and meet people. It manages at least two immune system enhancers simultaneously, as it will exercise and develop relationships at the same time. Many colleges and universities offer surprisingly cheap health and fitness programs.
5. Gadget lovers can purchase an exercise machine, such as a stair-climbing machine, a treadmill, and cross-country ski equipment, an exercise bike, or a Nautilus.
6. Turn a friend into an exercise buddy. Sometimes having a partner can only be the incentive needed to move forward.

7. Dance is aerobic, romantic, and social. There are many discos for counter dance, square dance, and swing that offer lessons and social connections.
8. Join a nature and hiking club, another way to combine exercise with social needs. The added benefits are numerous: you can be outdoors in nature, an excellent stress balancer; you will learn and become intimate with the natural world, and you will gain the confidence that comes from that knowledge. The earth supports us, but only by exploring the universe can we get to know this extraordinary truth.
9. Adult education programs abound in gymnastics classes, from aerobics and stretching to tai chi chuan and martial arts.

CHAPTER NINE
UNDERSTANDING THE STRESS CONNECTION TO THE BODY DEFENSES

The scenario is too familiar: you have to face an awkward situation, which will have a dramatic impact on your life and perhaps the lives of others. The day to day task of the company that determines its success or failure lies on your shoulders. Apply all your skills, hope for the best, but fear the worst. In the meantime, the dark possibilities of what could happen take advantage of his mind. You wake up late, worrying about the many variables that can affect the outcome. Maybe you lose some sleep. Physical symptoms arise shortness of breath and nervous tension in the arms, hands, and stomach. Your heartbeats and can even beat; A general feeling of confusion and doubt arises. It's called stress. When it persists for weeks or months, it is called chronic stress. It changes everything in your external environment and also a lot of what happens inside you.

The study of how stress affects the immune system, a science called psychoneuroimmunology, is among the most exciting areas of health research. Stress has a significant effect on the body's immune functions, and the impact of stress on immunity demonstrates the power each of us has on our health. It is possible to remove a massive load from the immune system and strengthen the immune response by reducing or eliminating stress.

Most of us experience problems from time to time. Those of us who have chronic discomfort, which means that we continually depress our immune system, increase our chances of getting sick. Stress increases the chance of getting a bacterial infection and a virus, including the common cold. It also increases the chances of serious degenerative diseases, such as heart disease, hypertension, cancer, asthma, diabetes, and inflammatory bowel disease. Many doctors believe that stress plays a role in the onset of multiple sclerosis, rheumatoid arthritis, and other autoimmune disorders, although these links have not yet been demonstrated. However, science has shown that stress is a depressant to the immune system, which means it puts us at risk of suffering from all kinds of ailments.

STRESS AND THE IMMUNE SYSTEM

A variety of immune functions are affected by stress. Recently, a team of researchers conducted a meta-analysis or overview of the best research in a specific field. After examining thirty-eight well-controlled studies examining the effects of stress on the immune system, scientists concluded that stress consistently reduces various types of immune responses. The immune system is simply weaker in people under pressure.

People who are under stress and therefore receive an antigen have lower immune responses than those who are not under pressure. Furthermore, natural killer cells decrease in number and activity in those under stress; In one study, the changes in cellular activity paralleled the changes in adrenaline. The higher the levels of adrenaline, the lower the responses of natural killer cells to a virus or cancer cell.

Research has also shown that cytokine production, such as interleukin-2 and interferon-gamma, also decreases with stress. This suggests that CD4 cells and macrophages are not functioning optimally (since they produce cytokines). The overall immune response will be weaker without sending these chemical messengers. The antibodies produced by B cells to fight the herpes virus tend to increase when people with herpes are under stress. As we pointed out in chapter 2, infections such as herpes and HIV can hide inside the cells, where they remain dormant until the immune system weakens, at which point the virus launches an attack.

The immune system responds in part by producing antibodies to fight the virus. The struggle occurs. But the battle has come in large part because the strength of the immune system has decreased, giving the virus a chance to get out of the hiding place, start replicating and get a higher position in the body.

Several studies report that the ratio of CD4 cells to CD8 cells decreases very often because the number of CD8 cells (immunosuppressants) increases.

EXAMS, STRESS, AND DEPRESSION OF THE IMMUNE SYSTEM

Ronald Glaser and Janice Kiecolt-Glaser, two longtime psychoneuroimmunology workers, have conducted a series of experiments over several years to examine the effects of test stress on medical students at Ohio State University. Each year, they monitor students' immune responses at times of reduced stress and during periods of high pressure immediately before the test. Not surprisingly, the researchers found that exam stress is associated with a decrease in general immunity. Several specific immune responses have been weakened, including T cells and natural killer cells and the production of interleukin-2 and interferon-gamma. The researchers also found an increase in antibodies to the Epstein-Barr virus, which means that during times of high stress, the virus had emerged from its hiding places inside the tissues.

Other researchers have also documented changes in the immune response to everyday tasks such as arithmetic tests and stressful interviews. In all these experiments, the observations have been consistent: low activity of natural killer cells and low immune response to a challenge. The effect of stress on the immune system occurs quickly. Weakened immune responses were observed within thirty minutes of taking the test or interview. Groups subject to other stressful life events, such as skydiving or pending the outcome of an HIV test, experienced poor immune function.

STRESS HAS AN INDEPENDENT EFFECT

Skeptics claim that stress does not have an independent effect; instead, it encourages people to increase behaviors that weaken the immune system, such as sleep loss, poor nutrition, smoking, excessive alcohol consumption, and other health-related actions. However, this argument has been proven false.

Glaser and Kiecolt-Glaser considered other possibilities for students' immune system depression, such as lack of sleep or lack of nutrition. They found that stress had an independent impact on immunity. When they looked at the effect of these factors independently, they found that changes in immune function were not related to changes in sleep or weight or changes in blood protein levels that would indicate malnutrition. Stress was debilitating on its own.

In another carefully controlled study, 154 men and 266 women were exposed to a virus, and therefore, the development of cold was monitored. There was a striking linear correlation between the amount of stress reported by subjects in the previous year and their susceptibility to colds. This study, as well as laboratory research, offered convincing evidence that common stress-related behaviors are not the cause of the observed changes in the immune response.

HORMONES AND STRESS

Stress, as many of us know firsthand, can wreak havoc on our hormones, which can have profound effects on our health. Some stress-related hormones directly contribute to cardiovascular disease. Some of these same hormones also create immune system dysfunction. Stress triggers the overproduction of a variety of neurochemicals. Among the most carefully studied is cortisol, a hormone produced by the adrenal glands. Cortisol prevents excessive use of energy in the event of a crisis. It also inhibits almost all aspects of the immune system. Stress increases cortisol production, which in turn reduces the immune response across the board.

Catecholamines, which include epinephrine (also called adrenaline) and noradrenaline (a neurotransmitter that, like adrenaline, also causes physical and emotional arousal), often cause intense physical sensations that we experience under stress, excess energy, rapid breathing and heart rate improved and physical coordination. Depending on the amount of these neurochemical substances in the blood, they grow or interfere with the communication between the receptors of an immune cell and the nucleus of the cell. Unfortunately, whenever we are under stress, especially for prolonged periods, these chemicals generally interfere with that communication. They, therefore, prevent immune cells from responding to antigens. Thus, hormonal imbalance weakens the immune response.

In addition to its effects on the immune system, stress is believed to contribute to the development of heart disease, asthma, ulcers, inflammatory bowel syndrome, diabetes, migraine, and premenstrual syndrome.

HUMANS VERSUS ANIMALS: WE ARE NOT THE BEST ADAPTERS

Humans are much more vulnerable to long-term or chronic stress, the more debilitating type, than other members of the animal kingdom. In animal studies, repeated exposure to stress, such as electric shock, causes the animal to adapt to stress so that it loses its immunosuppressive effect over time.

However, in human studies, the deterioration of the immune response tends to persist, especially when the source of stress is interpersonal. This means that it is not necessarily under the control of a single person. Sometimes human responses to chronic stress can be maladaptive. For example, the body typically has an integrated monitoring system that can disable additional production of cortisol, a hormone that depresses immunity, provided that cortisol levels are too high. However, when chronic depression arises, the monitoring system becomes inefficient so that cortisol continues to be produced in excess.

Humans also show a marked propensity to become overly sensitive to stress, so even the mere suggestion of a particular stressor, such as the bell of Pavlov's experiments, triggers a physical and, in this case, depressing response to immunity. For example, cancer patients who have undergone chemotherapy often experience nausea or vomiting whenever they anticipate or approach their next appointment for another cycle of medications. Parallel changes occur in the immune system. Women with ovarian cancer, for example, have experienced a reduced lymphocyte response as the next chemotherapy appointment approaches.

This same phenomenon occurs in other contexts where people experience long-term stress. For example, those who care for people living with Alzheimer's and women who have recently divorced or remain in unhappy marriages exhibit a compromised immune response. In particular, natural killer cells weaken and, if the virus is present, the antibodies against herpes increase. Such conditions make people more sensitive to a wide range of viral and bacterial diseases and cancer.

STRESS AND PRENATAL CONSIDERATIONS

Unfortunately, psychological stress during pregnancy can have lasting effects on offspring. The developing baby's brain is affected by abnormal neurochemicals and hormones when the mother is under pressure. Probably due to these developmental changes, the child's immune response weakens or deteriorates. Studies have shown that B cells and the antibodies they produce are particularly affected.

EUSTRESS AND DISTRESS

Like beauty, there are stressful situations in the eye of the beholder. A person can perceive challenges at home or work as opportunities to improve relationships, achieve personal goals, and use essential skills.

This person is more likely to enter the fray and, despite the difficulties, often finds himself appreciating the process. You have a little freedom to express yourself, take risks, and give yourself the freedom of experimentation and creativity. Therefore, he strengthens himself in the face of difficulties and exercises some control, which, as we will see in the next chapter, can improve immunity. On the contrary, another person perceives problems as a threat to their survival. He gives up on the challenge, plays it safe, and worries about the outcome of the events.

At some level, you realize that you have little or no power over the situation because you have withdrawn from the challenge. This, of course, will influence the quality of your efforts, both at home and at work, and will undoubtedly determine the outcome of the events. More importantly, it will significantly affect the quality of your life.

The first person is experiencing what scientists call eustress or the perception that the opportunity is in the challenge. This perception is based on the belief that the problematic situation's outcome will most likely be positive. Attitudes to the immune system are implicit in industry. The other person experiences anxiety, characterized by worry, anxiety, and fear. The anguish arises from the belief that the result of the problematic situation will be negative. Anguish depresses the immune system and can easily cause disease.

Ironically, two people facing the same situation may experience eustress while the other experiences distress.

In other words, our attitudes often determine whether an event is demanding or distressing. Fortunately, our moods can change.

Science is learning that, with the help of an impressive variety of techniques, you can transform your way of thinking and behaving to avoid the adverse effects of stress. Not only can it alter the quality of your life known since the birth of religion, but such changes can drastically increase your immune defenses. Here are some practical ways to do it.

MENTAL DRIVERS TO DRIVE YOUR IMMUNE SYSTEM

All of the following techniques help reduce stress and its adverse side effects. Many of them not only prevent immune depression but increase immune responses. However, some of the methods we offer have not been individually tested for their effects on immunity. However, if we agree that excessive stress damages the immune system (a well-known fact) and that reducing excess weight has a protective effect on immunity, it follows that established techniques for relaxation and stress management will, at least, have a protective effect the immune system.

PRAY, MEDITATE OR REPEAT A MANTRA

Nothing relaxes us like faith, and its effectiveness has been demonstrated several times in the laboratory.

Researchers from the University Of Miami Medicine School have found that daily meditation or relaxation exercises, or the gradual release of tension in the muscles of the whole body, increase CD4 cells. The study was conducted on men with HIV who typically exhibit a constant decline in CD4 cells. When Gail Ironson, MD, a psychiatrist at the University of Miami School of Medicine, and his colleagues followed the men a year later, they found that those men who continued to do some form of daily meditation or relaxation exercises were less likely suffer from AIDS symptoms.

Other research has shown that meditation or relaxation exercises have increased the activity of immune cells when challenged. One study showed an increase in natural killer cells and an increase in lymphocyte proliferation in medical students who practice a daily relaxation regimen.

"There are many forms of relaxation or meditation exercises," says Dr. Ironson. "They can be as simple as muscle relaxation, or meditate in a beautiful place in nature, or repeat a single word (like a mantra) over and over again in your head. We don't have enough data to distinguish the effects of each of these practices on the immune system. Still, research so far suggests that all of them, if practiced regularly, appear to have a positive impact. "

Harvard University psychologist Ellen Langer has discovered that Transcendental Meditation (TM) is a technique in which a person silently repeats a word or mantra, repeatedly, induces a profound state of relaxation and can be associated with greater longevity. After three years of study, Langer found that nursing home residents who practiced TM lived longer than those who didn't. All nursing home residents who practiced TM were still alive after three years of study, compared to a 38% mortality rate among patients who did not use the technique.

Herbert Benson, M.D., associate professor of medicine at Harvard Medical School, studied the effects of prayer and meditation on health thoroughly and found that such methods create what Benson calls the "response to relaxation." Benson says that a meditation session of ten to twenty minutes a day lowers blood pressure, lowers heart rate, relaxes muscles, and creates a more balanced hormonal condition, which can contribute to a more robust immune response.

USE A PROGRESSIVE RELAXATION TECHNIQUE

Like meditation, progressive relaxation techniques can change hormone levels, causing a decrease in the immunosuppressive hormone cortisol by increasing the hormone dehydroepiandrosterone sulfate, which boosts immunity. One study found that relaxation training increased the overall immune response in nursing home patients.

Another experiment found that relaxation triggered increased natural killer cell activity and lymphocyte proliferation in medical students undergoing testing, usually a situation that depresses the immune system.

A study found that the combined effects of relaxation techniques, exercise, and stress management increased T cells by 10 percent in a group of men infected with HIV. Another study reported that relaxation techniques, combined with dietary change and light exercise, were effective in lowering blood pressure like drug treatment, except that the change in behavior had the added benefit. To improve energy and sexual satisfaction.

MEDITATION

Try to meditate twice a day to relieve stress and deepen spirituality. The following reflection is an example of a progressive relaxation technique that many people have used successfully.

Lay comfortably on your back. Breathe rhythmically and deeply in a relaxed way. Visualize your feet, stretch your fingers and toes, and then relax suddenly. Do the same for the calves: visualize the calves' muscles, tighten them, and relax them suddenly. Do the same in sequence for the thighs, buttocks, stomach, chest, shoulders, hands, forearms, biceps, neck, and face. This meditation will create deep relaxation and relieve muscle tension and stress.

Do some variation in this exercise every day, and every time you are under stress.

BIOFEEDBACK TEST

Biofeedback may be the most effective technique for teaching people to achieve deep relaxation and to control tension and stress-related symptoms. In essence, the states of deep relaxation created during biofeedback sessions are the same as those experienced in progressive relaxation and meditation. The only difference is that these conditions are achieved with technological devices that measure body temperature, sweat, heart rate, and other physical symptoms. People learn to control all these physical symptoms with the use of such equipment.

They see firsthand that they can reduce temperature, sweat, and heart rate with their minds, and in the process, they achieve deep relaxation and increased immunity.

Biofeedback has proven to be effective in treating a wide range of problems, including angina, anxiety, asthma, intestinal ailments, chronic pain, epilepsy, headache and migraine, hypertension, high cholesterol, insomnia, learning difficulties., muscle spasm, phobias, fast heartbeat, TMJ (temporomandibular dysfunction), and urinary problems.

JOIN A SUPPORT GROUP

Structured groups can focus on education, social support, relaxation training, or developing coping skills. At least two studies show better immune system function in people involved in support groups. In one study, group support for melanoma patients resulted in a reduction of anxiety and depression and a parallel increase in the immune response. The activity of natural killer cells has been notably improved. So it was survival rates. Support groups have also been shown to increase the longevity of people with cancer, especially women with breast cancer.

Researchers from Clark University in Worcester, Massachusetts, found that the mere fact that people adopted the facial expression of a particular mood created that mood in people themselves. Emotions of fear provoked feelings of anxiety and stress. The same consistency of emotion and expression occurred when the subjects of the study were asked to adopt expressions of anger, disgust, and sadness. On the contrary, when the researchers asked people to repeat the letter several times, and feelings of happiness were generated by making a face adopt a smile-like expression.

This research supports the old song that pushes us to "spread the sunlight all over the place and put on a happy face."

Nothing takes the stress away from a difficult situation better than humor. The wise cultivate fun as a way of dealing with life because, let's face it, a lot of experience is absurd.

CONSIDER THERAPY

Find a professional consultant who can help you express your feelings and develop new ways of dealing with stressful situations. Expressions of pain or anger alone have not been shown to improve mood or immune response. However, patients on therapy who are encouraged to express grief and anger as they learn new life-support behaviors have demonstrated significant improvement in mood.

TAKE A HOT BATH

Believe it or not, hot baths cause more than just a placebo effect. Hot water relaxes the muscles, improves circulation, and slightly warms the brain, which, according to scientists, calms the whole system. The water temperature should not exceed 102 degrees Fahrenheit. Excess heat can be shocking to the system, causing the muscles to contract by increasing circulation, an unhealthy combination. Submerge in the container for no more than fifteen minutes. (People with diabetes should avoid hot baths entirely.)

BREATHE DEEPLY

Dean Ornish, M.D., director of the Preventive Medicine Research Institute in Sausalito, California, says that "deep breathing is one of the simplest and most effective stress management techniques around." Ornish demonstrated the reversal of atherosclerosis in the coronary arteries, a historic step in medicine using a low-fat diet, light exercise, and stress management program. Ornish's stress management program focused primarily on deep breathing, mainly to relieve physical tension and yoga. Deep and long-lasting exhalation is particularly relaxing. It releases physical tension and creates a focused sensation that is noticeably free of anxiety.

BODYWORK

Work on the body, such as acupressure, massage therapy, and therapeutic touch, creates deep relaxation and positively influences biochemistry and some immune responses. Make sure you see a certified professional.

HYPNOSIS TEST

Like relaxation techniques, hypnosis can induce deep relaxation and improve biochemical conditions. If none of the other relaxation techniques appeal to you, try hypnosis.

EXERCISE THE FAR BLUE

Studies revealed that people who exercise enjoy better psychological health and higher self-esteem than those who don't. Exercise increases mood and reduces depression, anxiety, and stress. It can even create euphoria. It also lowers blood pressure, increases HDL (the type of cholesterol that protects against atherosclerosis), and strengthens cardiovascular function. (See chapter 8 for more information on exercise and the mind.) Exercise changes brain chemistry. Twenty minutes of operation causes the brain to secrete beta-endorphins, which relieve depression and create feelings of well-being and optimism.

Studies have shown that running can be useful in improving the psychological state of some psychotherapeutic techniques. A research conducted on the effect of exercise on people in a psychiatric hospital unit found that exercise significantly reduced depression, anxiety and increased feelings of success. Dorothy Harris, a sports psychologist, and professor at Pennsylvania State University, says that running twenty minutes three times a week can have a profound effect on mental attitude and health.

EAT FOR YOUR MIND AND AS WELL AS YOUR BODY

Each meal changes brain chemistry and mood, according to research conducted at the Massachusetts Institute of Technology. Researcher John D. Fernstrom, Ph.D., wrote that "it is becoming increasingly clear that brain chemistry and function can be affected by a single meal. In the short term, in well-fed individuals who consume reasonable amounts of food changes in food composition can quickly affect brain function."

According to MIT researchers, the carbohydrates found in whole grains and whole wheat bread stimulate the production of a chemical neurotransmitter called serotonin, which creates feelings of well-being and inner peace. Serotonin calms anxiety, focuses the mind, relieves depression, and produces deeper sleep. As carbohydrate intake increases, serotonin levels increase, along with all these positive emotions.

According to Judith J. Wurtman, Ph.D., another MIT scientist and pioneer in this field, "Those who eat relaxing foods [containing carbohydrates] report feeling more relaxed, more focused, less stressed, less distracted after the meal." After people ate carbohydrates, they reported that "feelings of stress and tension are relieved, and concentration is improved," says Dr. Wurtman.

On the other hand, the scientists found that foods rich in animal protein cause an increase in dopamine and norepinephrine. These two neurotransmitters increase readiness, responsiveness, and aggression. The more protein you eat, the lower your serotonin levels will be. Therefore, protein foods elevate neurotransmitters that compete with brain serotonin levels and ultimately decrease.

Regardless of the stress-reducing techniques, you incorporate into your lifestyle, you can be sure that this will benefit both your mental state and the physical fitness of your immune system.

BONUS- HOW TO MAKE YOUR HAND SANITIZERS

While the flu continues to deteriorate by the day, the emphasis is being put on one particular aspect of personal hygiene: keeping your hands clean. However, this clarion call for clean hands had a downside – may be expected – as it resulted in scalpers buying hand sanitizer supplies and reselling them at inflated prices. The prices of standard retail hand sanitizers at different locations across the country grew to the point of absurdity. Are you unable to find a hand sanitizer? It's easier to wash your hands with soap, but if you don't have soap and water, then hand sanitizer is the second-best option. Commercial hand sanitizer may get costly, and you might have to make your own with the scarcity of hand sanitizer. Creating your hand sanitizer is a quick method that involves a recipe that can be customized to your personal preferences.

BE READY FOR COLD & FLU SEASON

The tartness of the air! The crunch of leaves on trees! Autumn's sights and sounds are here! When your home rings with the first sneeze of the season, only one thing can be said: the cold and flu season is upon us. Let's work together to ensure that these nasty germs are kept at a low price by producing an all-natural hand sanitizer.

HAND SANITIZER: RECIPE 1

Most of the DIY Sanitizer Recipes you have come across do not work – This is the best way to do it.

Materials required (small volume production)

REAGENTS FORMULATION 1

- Ethanol 96%: 8333ml
- Hydrogen peroxide 3%: 417ml
- Glycerol 98%: 145ml
- Sterile distilled or boiled cold water

REAGENT FORMULATION 2

- Isopropyl Alcohol 99.8%: 7515ml
- Hydrogen peroxide 3%: 417ml
- Glycerol 98%: 145ml
- Sterile distilled or boiled cold water

MATERIALS FOR DIY HAND SANITIZER

- 10-liter plastic or glass bottles with threaded stoppers, or
- 50-liter plastic containers (mostly the ones made with polypropylene or high-density polyethylene, translucent to see the liquid level), or
- Stainless steel tanks with a capacity of 80 –100 liters (used for the mixing process to avoid wastage)
- Paddles made of wood, plastic or metal for mixing
- Calibrated cylinders and jugs
- Funnel made of Plastic or metal
- 100 ml Plastic bottles with tops that are leakproof
- 500 ml plastic or glass bottles with tops that are screwed
- An alcoholometer: To measure the quantity of alcohol in the mixture.

IMPORTANT THINGS TO KEEP IN MIND

Glycerol: used as a humectant; however, it can also be used with other skincare emollients, provided it is inexpensive, widely available, and miscible in water and alcohol.

Hydrogen peroxides are used in the solution for inactive bacterial contaminating spores and are not active ingredients for antiseptic handling.

Any additional additives for both formulations must be clearly labeled and non-toxic in case of accidental consumption.

To allow distinction with other fluids, a colorant can be added but must not be toxic, encourage allergy, or contain antimicrobial properties. It is not suggested to add perfumes or colors, due to the possibility of allergic reactions.

METHOD OF PREPARATION

As stated above, we can use a 10-liter plastic bottle to mix the ingredients.

PREPARATION INSTRUCTIONS:

1. The alcohol used for the solution is poured into the large bottle or tank to the graduation point, as shown below.

2. The measuring cylinder is used to add hydrogen oxide.

3. The glycerol is mixed in the solution with the help of a measuring cylinder. Since glycerol is very acidic and stains the surface of the measuring container, it can be rinsed with distilled water or cold boiled water and then poured into the tank.

4. Then the tank is filled with distilled water or cold boiled water up to the limit of 10 liters.

5. After preparation, the cap or screw cap is mounted as soon as possible on the tank/bottle, to avoid evaporation. After preparation, the cap or the cap of the crew is mounted as soon as possible on the tank/bottle, to avoid evaporation. (Both 4 and 5 are described below)

6. The solution is stirred by gentle shaking or using a scoop, if necessary.

7. Distribute the solution into its final containers (for example, 500 ml or 100 ml plastic bottles) and quarantine the battles for 12 hours before use. This allows you to remove the spores present in alcohol or new / reused bottles.

LABEL GUIDELINES AND INFORMATION

Labeling should be consistent with national standards, and must include:

- Institution Name
- Recommended hand rubs formulation by WHO
- For external use only
- Avoid contact with eyes
- Keep out of the reach of children

- Date of production and batch number
- Usage: Apply a palm-full of alcohol-based hand rub and cover all surfaces of the hands until it is dry.
- Composition: glycerol, hydrogen peroxide, ethanol, or isopropanol.
- Flammable: Don't store close to fire or heat

HAND SANITIZER: RECIPE 2

Learn how to make natural and easy DIY Hand sanitizer. This hand-made sanitizer works well, saves money, and helps fight cold and flu!

The essential oil you use can also help protect you against germs and add fragrance to your hand sanitizer. Thyme and clove oil, for example, have antimicrobial properties. When using antimicrobial oils, use just one or two drops, as these oils appear to be very strong and can irritate your skin. Other oils, including chamomile or lavender, can help soothe your skin.

WHAT YOU'LL NEED
1. Equipment / tools
- bowl and spoon
- Funnel
- Bottle with pump distributor

2. Materials
- 2/3 cup of 99% isopropyl alcohol
- (isopropyl alcohol) or ethanol
- 1/3 cup of aloe vera gel
- 1/4 teaspoon of vitamin E oil (helps soften hands!)
- 30 drops tea tree essential oil

None of it could be simpler! Just whisk the ingredients together and then pour them into the container using the funnel. Screw the pump into the bottle again, and you're good to go.

3. Steps to Follow

- In a small ceramic bowl or cup, add essential oils and vitamin E oil and mix well;
- Combine the oils with alcohol, and blend again.
- Stir the mixture with the aloe vera gel and mix well.
- Shake gently before use.
- Transfer the hand sanitizer to small, clean squirt bottles.
- Also, use colored bottles like this so that the essential oils in the recipe are not exposed to light.
- This recipe is perfect for throwing in a purse or a bag at the end of the day!

Notes:

To make a hand sanitizer spray, use witch hazel instead of an aloe vera gel in this recipe.

Important tips and warnings about this recipe

In the recipe, lavender is used to reduce the strong odor of tea tree oil. If you are not a lavender addict, choose antibacterial oil, such as rosemary, sage, sandalwood, or peppermint.

Always take care of the handling of essential oils. They are very concentrated, potent plant extracts. If you're new to using essential oils, you may want to test for any allergic reaction before slathering on this homemade hand sanitizer. Like any natural plant, the family members may be allergic. Combine a drop of the essential oil with one tablespoon of olive oil for a simple patch test.

Apply some on the inside of your elbow, cover it with a bandage, and wait for twenty-four hours to see if there is any negative reaction. If you have read recent studies about how dangerous the use of hand sanitizers can be, bear in mind that the danger is present in the chemicals used in industrial sanitizers. This handmade sanitizer recipe does not include those harmful chemicals and depends on pure essential oils to kill germs. Some of the special advantages of essential oils are that they do not induce bacterial resistance such as antibacterial agents, and are actually effective in destroying bacterial species that have become immune to our man-made medicines and agents.

Sometimes enabling our bodies to encounter germs and improve our immune systems is fine, but also having a hand sanitizer available for emergencies is better. In these situations, this gentle homemade hand sanitizer is one of the better alternatives to commercial products.

COMPOSITION OF IN-HOUSE / LOCAL ALCOHOL-BASED FORMULATIONS

The preference WHO hand rubs component takes into account both expense constraints and microbiological effectiveness. Procurement of raw ingredients will be affected by market availability of under standard materials, and careful selection of local sources is necessary. For preparation in- house or at a nearby production plant, the following two alcohol-based hand rub formulations are recommended, up to a limit of 50 liters:

Formulation No 1: Glycerol 1.45 percent v / v. Hydrogen peroxide (H_2O_2) 0.125 percent v/ v, to obtain final concentrations of ethanol 80 percent v/v.

Formulation No2: For the processing of final concentrations of isopropyl alcohol 75 percent v/v, glycerol 1.45 percent v/ v, hydrogen peroxide

(H_2O_2) 0.125 percent v/ v: only reagents of pharmacopeia standard (e.g., International Pharmacopoeia) should be used and not products of technical grade.

PRODUCTION AND STORAGE

The creation of WHO-approved hand rub formulation is feasible at centralized dispensaries or pharmacies. Governments should promote local production, endorse the quality assurance process, and keep production costs as small as possible, where feasible and in line with local policies. Special specifications apply to the manufacture and storage of products, as well as to raw material storage.

Cleansing and disinfection process for reusable hand rub bottles:

1. Bring empty bottles to a location central reprocessing via normal operating protocols;

2. To remove any leftover fluids, wash bottles thoroughly with detergent and tap-water;

3. If it resists heat, disinfect bottles by boiling in water. Thermal disinfection should be preferred over chemical disinfection, whenever possible. The latter can increase costs and require an additional phase to flush the disinfectant's remains out. Chemical disinfection should include soaking the bottles for at least 15 minutes in a solution containing 10XX) ppm of chlorine, and afterward rinsing with sterile boiling water;

After chemical or thermal disinfection, place the bottles in a bottle rack to dry absolutely upside down. The dry bottles should be covered with a lid and stored before use, safe from dust.

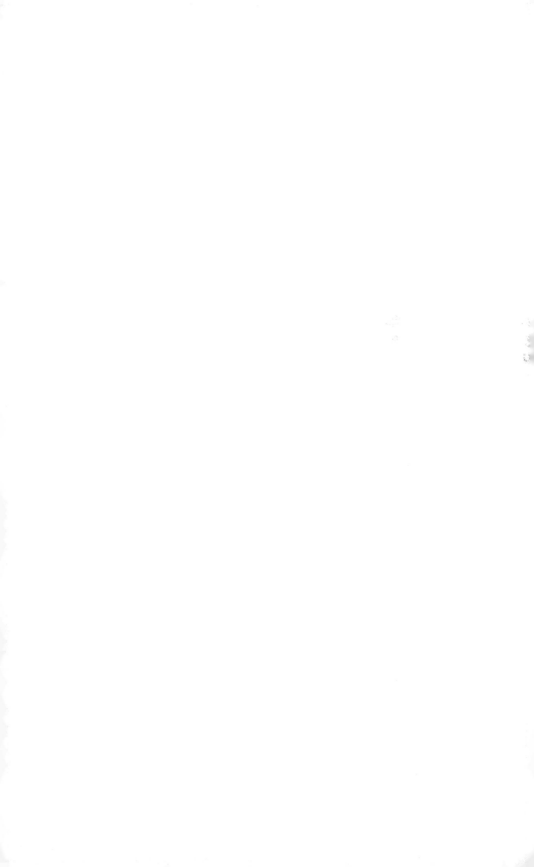

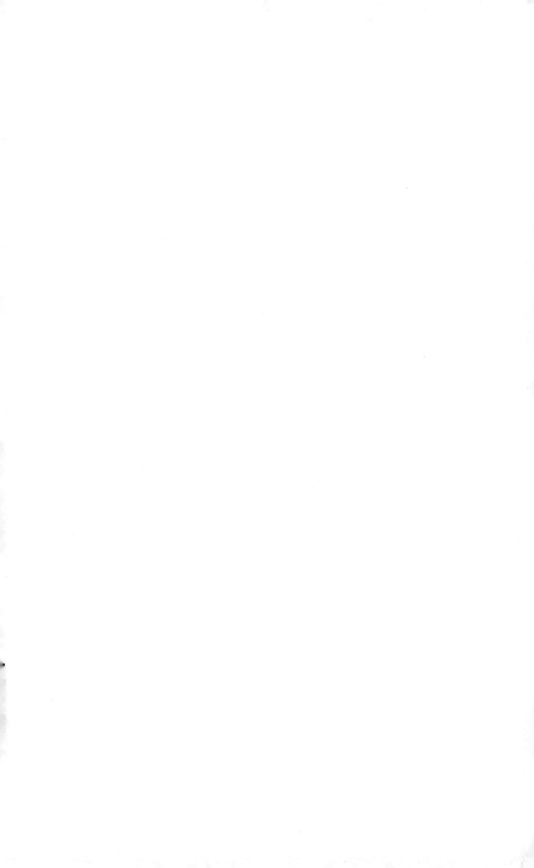

Made in the USA
Columbia, SC
09 September 2020